Electronic Prescribing

A Safety and Implementation Guide

Michael Van Ornum, RPh, RN, BCPS
Chair, Joint Physician Pharmacy Group
Secretary, Pharmacy Society of Rochester
Consulting Clinical Pharmacist, GRIPA

D0555618

JONES AND BARTLETT PUBLISHERS
Sudbury, Massachusetts
BOSTON   TORONTO   LONDON   SINGAPORE

World Headquarters

Jones and Bartlett Publishers
40 Tall Pine Drive
Sudbury, MA 01776
978-443-5000
info@jbpub.com
www.jbpub.com

Jones and Bartlett Publishers
Canada
6339 Ormindale Way
Mississauga, Ontario L5V 1J2
Canada

Jones and Bartlett Publishers
International
Barb House, Barb Mews
London W6 7PA
United Kingdom

Jones and Bartlett's books and products are available through most bookstores and online booksellers. To contact Jones and Bartlett Publishers directly, call 800-832-0034, fax 978-443-8000, or visit our website www.jbpub.com.

Substantial discounts on bulk quantities of Jones and Bartlett's publications are available to corporations, professional associations, and other qualified organizations. For details and specific discount information, contact the special sales department at Jones and Bartlett via the above contact information or send an email to specialsales@jbpub.com.

The authors, editor, and publisher have made every effort to provide accurate information. However, they are not responsible for errors, omissions, or for any outcomes related to the use of the contents of this book and take no responsibility for the use of the products and procedures described. Treatments and side effects described in this book may not be applicable to all people; likewise, some people may require a dose or experience a side effect that is not described herein. Drugs and medical devices are discussed that may have limited availability controlled by the Food and Drug Administration (FDA) for use only in a research study or clinical trial. Research, clinical practice, and government regulations often change the accepted standard in this field. When consideration is being given to use of any drug in the clinical setting, the health care provider or reader is responsible for determining FDA status of the drug, reading the package insert, and reviewing prescribing information for the most up-to-date recommendations on dose, precautions, and contraindications, and determining the appropriate usage for the product. This is especially important in the case of drugs that are new or seldom used.

Production Credits

Publisher: David Cella
Acquisitions Editor: Kristine Johnson
Editorial Assistant: Maro Asadoorian
Production Director: Amy Rose
Production Editor: Renée Sekerak
Production Assistant: Julia Waugaman
Associate Marketing Manager: Lisa Gordon
Manufacturing and Inventory Control Supervisor:
    Amy Bacus

Assistant Print Buyer: Jessica DeMarco
Composition: Auburn Associates, Inc.
Photo Research Manager/Photographer: Kimberly Potvin
Cover Design: Brian Moore
Cover Image: © Photos.com
Printing and Binding: Malloy Incorporated
Cover Printing: Malloy Incorporated

Photo Credits

Figures E.3–E.8: Doctor, Nurse, Pharmacist, Customer Service Representative: © Roslen Mack/ShutterStock, Inc; Family: © Lorelyn Medina/ShutterStock, Inc.

Figure F.1: Checkbox: ©gnet2000/ShutterStock, Inc.; Compass: ©Bruce Rolff/ShutterStock, Inc.; Person: ©Roslen Mack/ShutterStock, Inc.; Paper: © Kluke/ShutterStock, Inc.; Mortar and pestle: ©Lidiya Drabchuk/ShutterStock, Inc.

Figure F.2: Checkbox: ©gnet2000/ShutterStock, Inc.; Prescription: ©TheSupe87/ShutterStock, Inc.; Computer: ©Feng Yu/ShutterStock, Inc.; Checkboxes: ©Anastasios Kandris/ShutterStock, Inc.; Life preserver: ©Slavoljub Pantelic/ShutterStock, Inc.

Figure F.3: Checkbox, Lightning Bolt: ©gnet2000/ShutterStock, Inc.; Graph: ©Pling/ShutterStock, Inc.; Star: ©Lindaphoto/ShutterStock, Inc.

Library of Congress Cataloging-in-Publication Data
Van Ornum, Michael.
    Electronic prescribing : a safety and implementation guide / by Michael Van Ornum.
        p. ; cm.
    Includes bibliographical references and index.
    ISBN 978-0-7637-5849-3 (pbk.)
    1. Internet pharmacies. 2. Drugs—Prescribing. 3. Pharmaceutical industry—Technological innovations. I. Title.
    [DNLM: 1. Prescriptions, Drug. 2. Decision Support Systems, Clinical. 3. Internet. QV 748 V217e 2009]
    RS122.2.V36 2009
    381'.45615102854678—dc22
6048   2008003028

Printed in the United States of America
12   11   10   09   08   10   9   8   7   6   5   4   3   2   1

*I would like to acknowledge my children,
who gave up a summer with their father, and my wife,
who patiently supported her husband's distraction.*

Contents

Reviewer Recognition

The author and the publisher would like to thank the following reviewers for their assistance in preparing this publication.

Andrew Case MS, RPA-C
Clinical Instructor
D'Youville College PA Program

Bruce W. Chaffee, PharmD

Jesse A. Coale, PA-C
Assistant Professor
Physician Assistant Program
Philadelphia University

Maria Friedman, DBA

Kim Galt, PharmD
Professor of Pharmacy Practice
Associate Dean for Research
Director, Creighton Health Services Research Program (CHRP)
School of Pharmacy and Health Professions
Creighton University

Jeffery A. Goad, PharmD, MPH, FCPhA, FCSHP
Associate Professor of Clinical Pharmacy
School of Pharmacy
University of Southern California

Michael Koncilja, RPh

Deb Lange, MS
Director, Analysis
Greater Rochester Independent Practice Association

Ann Llewellyn, RN, CMM
Practice Manager
Northgate Medical Group

Sam Mahrous, PhD, MBA
Midwestern University
College of Pharmacy–Glendale
Associate Professor
Arizona College of Medicine

Ken Majkowski, PharmD
Vice President
Clinical Affairs and Product Strategy
RxHub LLC

Eric T. Nielsen, MD
Greater Rochester Independent Practice Association

Richard O'Brocta, PharmD
Director of Experiential Education
Wegmans School of Pharmacy
St. John Fisher College

Roger M. Oskvig, MD
University of Rochester School of Medicine and Dentistry

Michael T. Rupp, PhD, RPh
Professor of Pharmacy Administration
Midwestern University–Glendale

Ranjit Singh, MA, MB, BChir (Cantab.), MBA
Assoc. Director, Patient Safety
Research Center Medical Director, Skilled Nursing Facility Assistant
Professor of Clinical Family Medicine School of Medicine and
Biomedical Sciences State University of New York at Buffalo

Marie Smith, PharmD
Dept. Head and Clinical Professor–Pharmacy Practice
University of Connecticut School of Pharmacy

Joseph M. Waltz, RPh MBA
Pharmacy Society of Rochester

Cori Wyman, PharmD, CDE

Preface

Health Care in Crisis

In 1999, the Institute of Medicine released a landmark report that indicated medical errors in the United States claim 44,000 to 98,000 lives each year, an amount greater than breast cancer or AIDS. Electronic prescribing has been identified as a large part of the solution,[2] and in February of 2007, **Allscripts** made its electronic prescribing program, **eRx NOW**, freely available to all prescribers.[3] Does ready access to e-prescribing represent a mortal blow to medication errors, or is more work required?[4,5]

Electronic prescribing, or e-prescribing, is the communication of prescription information between the prescriber's computer and the pharmacist's computer.[6] It is a tool that drives efficiency in the physician's office, increases patient satisfaction, reduces the time it takes a pharmacist to process a prescription,[7-9] and eliminates a large number of errors generated by paper systems.[10-12] E-prescribing makes renewing multiple prescriptions a task of seconds instead of half an hour.[13] Office phones don't ring as often.[14] The time between paper refills in the fax machine goes longer and longer. But e-prescribing is not a panacea.[15] Studies have shown that implementation of electronic prescribing doesn't eliminate errors; rather, the type of error changes.[16] Like any tool, its usefulness depends on how it is applied.[17-19]

Adoption of electronic prescribing inserts a fundamental change in the physician practice that affects the staff, patients, and pharmacies.[20] Electronic prescribing is more than a technology; it's a different way of managing business as usual. Successfully bridging the gap to this new way of practice requires an understanding of the technology, sensitivity to the effects of implementation on office staff and their roles, and awareness of the impact the technology has on patient safety.[1,21] We must understand the systems around us to provide safe, efficient patient care in today's increasingly complex healthcare environment.

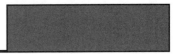

Introduction

Why Read This Book?

If you work with prescriptions or medical orders, chances are very good you will be managing these electronically in the near future, if you're not already. Many errors seen with paper prescriptions take a different form when recast as electronic prescriptions.[1] Whether you are a nurse, physician, office manager, or medical secretary, this book can give you the information you need to use electronic prescribing safely, to help you understand how e-prescribing works, to recognize what e-prescribing features can help or hinder safe prescribing, and to give you practical advice for implementing e-prescribing.

How to Use This Book

E-prescribing involves multiple disciplines; any discussion of implementation that ignores the effects of a prescriber's choice on a pharmacist, nurse, or patient would be incomplete—a multidisciplinary awareness is critical for patient safety. In deference to this, sidebars inserted throughout the book contrast the concerns of pharmacists with those of the medical office.

The New E-Prescriber

The new e-prescriber may be a nurse, physician, physician assistant, or other individual involved with creating or renewing prescriptions who now needs to use e-prescribing. The new e-prescriber needs information to use

(continues)

The New E-Prescriber *(continued)*

e-prescribing safely and effectively on a daily basis. Readers in this group should begin with Part I: Foundations, to gain the proper frame of reference. From there, consider:

- All the chapters of Part II to understand the capabilities and functions of e-prescribing in more detail.

- Chapter 7 to understand clinical decision support.

- Chapter 9 to understand the patient safety issues with e-prescribing and ways to prevent errors.

This book is designed for the clinician in everyday practice and maintains a focus on patient safety throughout. At times, a discussion of regulatory issues such as Health Insurance Portability and Accountability Act (HIPAA), administrative issues such as vendor contracting, and technical issues such as complex information technology configurations could be expanded. Appropriate references are noted where these topics exceed the scope of the book.

The E-Prescribing Purchaser/Evaluator

The person responsible for evaluating and making the final decision on e-prescribing–capable software is the e-prescribing purchaser.

- Chapter 8: Evaluating E-Prescribing Applications, provides detailed information from a clinician's perspective. This is also a useful section to review if the clinician is asked to evaluate an e-prescribing–capable application.

- If more background information is needed the purchaser or evaluator should read Part II: The Tools, Chapters 6 and 7, and Part IV: Implementation, which provide a good sense of operations and workflow needs. Considerations such as contracting, support negotiations, HIPAA security, and other factors involved in making a decision to purchase are beyond the scope of this book.

Professionals will interact with e-prescribing on a variety of levels. Some professionals may be new to the technology entirely while others are looking to upgrade a healthcare application that includes e-prescribing functions. Still others may be looking for further insight into this technology. The chapters in the book are designed to be semi-independent of one another. Prescribers, pharmacists, and others can find and read the sections most appropriate to their situation—the book does not have to be read from front to back. As a result of this approach, there is a small amount of redundancy between chapters, though internal references eliminate the need to repeat large sections of text.

The Implementer

The person responsible for training staff, developing workflows in the office, and making the transition to e-prescribing as smooth as possible benefits most from Part IV: Implementation. This is also true when making a substantial upgrade from one system to another. If more detail is needed:

- Chapter 2 provides background information on e-prescribing's infrastructure.

- Part II, Chapters 6 and 7 provide detailed information on functions that may affect implementation.

A scale in the beginning of each chapter indicates the general relevance of the chapter to prescribers, pharmacists, office managers, e-prescribing program designers, and nurse/medical assistants as follows:

Essential: This chapter contains information particularly suited to the profession or role.

Suggested: This chapter contains information generally suited to the profession or role.

Supplemental: This chapter provides information of general interest or historical in nature.

Other features are highlighted where appropriate in the following manner:

 This symbol identifies specific examples that can be used when evaluating or testing an e-prescribing program.

 This symbol indicates an increase in **communication** and corresponding benefit to patient safety.

 This symbol indicates a decrease in **communication** and corresponding risk to patient safety.

 This symbol indicates an increase in **complexity** and corresponding risk to patient safety.

This symbol indicates a decrease in **complexity** and corresponding benefit to patient safety.

The appendices contain forms and tools relevant to different aspects of electronic prescribing safety and implementation. A glossary of key terms is included at the back of the book; the terms are bolded on first reference in the text to allow easy access to the context and use of the term.

The Safety-Conscious User

Some clinicians may already be using e-prescribing and wish to improve their efficiency and/or decrease the potential for error. Chapter 9: E-Prescribing Safely, is the best place to start. From there, clinicians should consider:

- Chapters 2, 6, 7, and all of Part II for a more detailed understanding of e-prescribing safety issues.

PART I

Foundations

Myth Perceptions

READING PRIORITY

Definitions

Electronic prescribing (e-prescribing, e-Rx)—A type of computer technology whereby physicians use handheld or personal computer devices to review drug and formulary coverage and to transmit prescriptions to a printer or to a local pharmacy. E-prescribing software can be integrated into existing clinical information systems to allow physician access to patient-specific information to screen for drug interactions and allergies.[22]

Electronic prescription (e-prescription)—Refers to prescription information that is created, stored, and transmitted via electronic means by computer or handheld device. The term *electronic prescriptions* would not apply to prescriptions communicated either by facsimile (fax) or over the phone.[23]

A Very Brief History

Electronic prescribing traces its beginnings to the portable desktop assistants (PDAs) of the late 1980s and the 1990s. In 2003, the Medicare Modernization

Act charged the Centers for Medicare and Medicaid Service (**CMS**) with developing standards for electronic prescribing. In 2007, almost 25 years from the birth of e-prescribing, the first pilot of those standards has concluded.[24]

The effects on e-prescribing by the Health Insurance Portability and Accountability Act of 1996 (HIPAA)—which authorized the establishment of privacy and security safeguards for personal health information[25]—are significant, with the greatest challenge now centered on community-level integration of health information.[26] See also Chapter 6.

Frequently Asked Questions

This chapter addresses common preconceptions and concerns about e-prescribing before stepping into the subject directly. The following are a sampling of questions from pharmacists and physicians.

Questions about the Business Case

Question: Are pharmacies ready to receive electronic prescriptions?
Answer: Yes. More than 95% of the nation's pharmacies are certified for e-prescribing.[27] Inconsistent use of the terms *electronic prescription* and *electronic prescribing* by application **vendors**, pharmacists, doctors, and other healthcare professionals contributes to misperceptions regarding e-prescribing.

Many e-prescribing applications automatically determine if a pharmacy can receive the prescription electronically or by fax. As a result, the method of sending is transparent to the **prescriber**, though the safety profiles between the two methods are very different. See also Chapter 2.

Pharmacist Perspective

Local pharmacies should communicate their ability to receive electronic prescriptions to high-volume providers not using e-prescribing, especially those sending prescriptions as a computer-to-fax transmission. The provider might easily change to an **electronic data interchange (EDI)** format, but may need help to do so.[28] **SureScripts** has a fax communication for this purpose available for download at www.surescripts.com. Adoption of electronic prescribing and use of the EDI transaction significantly reduces the pharmacist's time spent entering prescriptions.[8,9]

Question: How much does e-prescribing cost?

Answer: E-prescribing has been sold to physicians under a variety of pricing models ranging from free to monthly subscription fees. In February of 2007, **Allscripts** made its e-prescribing application, **eRx NOW**, available at no cost to prescribers through the National ePrescribing Patient Safety Initiative (**NEPSI**).[3] Other free e-prescribing solutions may be available as part of an **electronic medical records (EMR)** package. Integrated health systems, **regional health information organizations (RHIOs)**, other **health information exchanges (HIEs)**, and local independent practice associations (IPAs) are also making electronic prescribing available at no cost to prescribers.

Though the application may be free, there are other costs to the prescriber. E-prescribing should be run on a current (within 2 years) desktop, laptop, or PDA with the vendor's suggested operating system. A high-speed internet connection is almost universally required. Paper, toner, and a printer are needed to print prescriptions. Staff time is invested in training. Patient visits may need to be rescheduled to allow the office time for implementation, which may affect office revenue. Staff time is needed to ensure patient medical histories are populated in the e-prescribing application. Some offices may require additional vendor support services and incur an additional fee.

Free applications may be more expensive than expected, but there is good news. Most of the expenses are front loaded with few ongoing obligations. Proper planning keeps those up-front costs to a minimum. See also Chapters 10, 11, and 12.

(R) Pharmacist Perspective

The direct cost of e-prescribing is painfully obvious to pharmacists both in the cost for the pharmacy dispensing application and in transaction fees. Like claims adjudication, a fee is charged on a per-transaction basis. Unlike claims adjudication, in which a fee is applied for every transaction, the pharmacy is only charged for the successful processing of a new e-prescription or e-renewal request. Subsequent pharmacy refills of an electronically received order do not trigger a charge; nor do incomplete transactions, whether initiated by the pharmacy or physician. See also Chapter 2.

Example: An electronic prescription for lisinopril 10 mg daily with five refills can be filled six times at the pharmacy. The initial fill generates an e-prescribing transaction charge while the subsequent five refills do not.

Question: Who makes money with e-prescribing?

Answer: The vendors of e-prescribing applications and services may be the only ones who actually generate revenue from e-prescribing. Pharmacies pay a fee for each electronic prescription transaction. The routing company that handles the transaction receives a portion of that fee, as does the e-prescribing application vendor and pharmacy application vendor.

Other people and institutions tend to enjoy cost savings as opposed to revenue. Insurers benefit when prevention of adverse drug events results in fewer hospitalizations,[29,30] when prescribers use more generic than brand-name drugs, and when fewer unnecessary tests are ordered. Some applications foster the use of clinical pathways, driving quality and cost-effectiveness that reduce general medical expenses. Patients benefit from lower co-pays associated with the generic drugs. Prescribers and pharmacists benefit from increased efficiency in the workplace.[31]

Because of these cost-saving benefits, insurance companies and government grants have, in the past, subsidized portions of the e-prescribing process for specific projects. Insurers bear much of the cost of making formulary and benefit content available to e-prescribing application vendors.

Question: Is e-prescribing technology stable or will my vendor disappear?

Answer: The technology is stable. E-prescribing is deeply embedded within the agendas of several national movements. The Institute of Medicine recommends that every prescriber and pharmacy use e-prescribing by 2010,[32] the Institute for Safe Medical Practices has called for the elimination of paper prescriptions,[10] the Joint Commission included electronic prescription records as part of its 2007 National Patient Safety Goals,[33] and CMS is overseeing the development of electronic prescribing standards.[24] Whether a vendor will be around to service its product is dependent on the health of the vendor company, not the technology of electronic prescribing.

SureScripts maintains a current list of e-prescribing vendors and pharmacies certified for e-prescribing transactions through the Pharmacy Health Information Exchange. For anyone who is in the market for an e-prescribing application, the SureScripts list **(Table 1.1)** is a good place to start looking.

Questions about Security

Question: Can a smart computer hacker use electronic prescribing to write prescriptions in my name for controlled substances?

Answer: No. Federal laws prohibit the electronic prescribing of controlled substances.[34] Standards to allow electronic prescribing are under consideration by the Drug Enforcement Agency (DEA)[34,35] and should be ready for industry implementation by the end of 2008. In the interim, the best practice

TABLE 1.1 SureScripts List in 2007

Company	Product
Allscripts	HealthMatics EMR 4.8.1
Allscripts	TouchWorks 10.1.1
Allscripts/NEPSI	eRx NOW 1.0
ASP.MD	ASP.MD
athenahealth	athenaClinicals
Axolotl	Elysium 8.0.1
Blue Cross and Blue Shield of Alabama	InfoSolutions 2.0
BMA Enterprises	Chart Management System 1.2
Bond Medical	Bond EHR Clinician 2006
Cerner	Health Record 3.0
Cerner	PowerChart M2007
ChartConnect	MedManager 6.8
Computer Programs and Systems, Inc. (CPSI)	Medical Practice 14
DAW Systems	ScriptSure
digiChart OB-GYN	digiChart 7.0
Doc-U-Chart	Doc-U-Scrip 4.0
DrFirst	DrFirst Rcopia 3.6.01
eClinicalWorks, Inc.	eClinicalWorks 7.0
Eclipsys	Sunrise Ambulatory Care Manager 4.5 XA
eHealthSolutions	eHealthSolutions 4.4
EHS	CareRevolution 5.1
e-MDs	e-MDs Solution Series 6.1
Epic	EpicCare EMR Spring 2007
Epic	EpicWeb Spring 2007
Gold Standard	eMPOWERx 3.09
H2H Solutions, Inc.	Digital Rx 1.5x
Henry Schein Medical Systems	MicroMD EMR 5.0
iMedica	Patient Relationship Manager 2007
iMedX	TurboRx
InstantDx	OnCallData 3.5

continues

TABLE 1.1 (continued)

Company	Product
InteGreat	IC-Chart 5.0
iSALUS	OfficeEMR
Kryptiq	Providing connectivity for GE Centricity EMR eScript Messenger 1.1
LighthouseMD	CareTracker 5.7
LSS Data Systems	Client Server 4
McKesson	Horizon Ambulatory Care 9.4.1
M.D. Web Solutions	AMCIS EMR 4.2AP.S
MedAppz	iSuite 3.5.000
MedComSoft	Record 2006/Ultimate Edition
MedConnect, Inc.	MedConnect EHR 1.0
Medent	MEDENT 17
Medical Communication Systems	mMD.net EMR 9.1
Medical Information Systems, Inc.	ChartMaker
MedicWare	MedicWare EMR 6.7
Medi-EMR	Medi-EMR
MediNotes	MediNotes EMR 5.2
MedNet System	emr4MD
MedPlexus	MedPlexus
MedPlus	Care360 Physician Portal 5.0
Misys	eScript 3.5
Misys	Misys EMR 8.10.1
NaviMedix	NaviNet 1.0.0.88
Netsmart-InfoScriber	InfoScriber
NewCrop	NewCrop 6.1
NextGen	NextGen EMR 5.5
OA Systems	Rx Cure 1.0
Polaris	EpiChart 5.0
Practice Partner	Practice Partner 9.2.1
Prematics	ScriptTone 2199

continues

TABLE 1.1 (continued)

Company	Product
Purkinje	CareSeries 2.0
RelayHealth	eScript 7.2
RxNT	EMR LITE 7.0
RxNT	RxNT 6.1.3
SOAPware	SOAPware 5.0
SSIMED	EMRge 6.0.57
SynaMed	SynaMed 4.0.040423
VipaHealth Solutions	SmartEMR 5.5
Waiting Room Solutions	Web Based EMR & Practice Management System 3.0
Wellogic	Consult 3.10.4
ZixCorp	PocketScript 6.7

Source: SureScripts List in 2007 (www.surescripts.com)

for e-prescribing users is to print out and sign every controlled substance prescription. You can send it to the pharmacy by fax, mail, or patient. Many e-prescribing applications will not allow the electronic transmission of a controlled substance prescription and will only display the print option. This is a desirable feature that protects the prescriber.

Delaying implementation of e-prescribing solely because of the laws around controlled substances is not warranted in most cases. In spite of the need to print prescriptions for controlled substances, e-prescribing still demonstrates significant safety and efficiency benefits.

 Pharmacist Perspective

If a prescription for a controlled substance appears on the fax machine without a signature, it is nonlegal.[36] Some e-prescribing applications will print words on the prescription similar to, "This prescription has been electronically signed," or it will print a logo or a seal. Consult your state laws about the acceptability of these prescriptions for noncontrolled substances.

(continues)

> **Pharmacist Perspective** *(continued)*
>
> Many states require special prescription paper for controlled substances with the letters *VOID* appearing on the prescription when it is copied or faxed. Absence of the VOID mark on a prescription implies a computer-to-fax transmission, which implies an e-prescribing application generated the transmission. Few offices routinely generate copies of their prescriptions for the patient's chart. Contact with the prescriber or office is needed to confirm that a follow-up, signed paper prescription is in the mail. Absence of the VOID may also indicate prescription fraud. Judgment is needed to differentiate between a valid prescription and fraud.
>
> The presence of the VOID mark implies a fax-to-fax transmission, which implies the prescription exists in paper form at the prescriber's office. The decision of whether to make the phone call to the prescriber in this circumstance is driven by pharmacist judgment and legal obligations.

Question: Can controlled substances be prescribed electronically after the federal government releases standards in 2008?

Answer: The DEA and industry disagree on the appropriate security for the transmission of controlled substance prescriptions.[35] The standards for transmitting electronic prescriptions have been in place and functional since 2001. Six years later, the most basic transactions allowed by the standards are still not found in all e-prescribing applications.[27] More time will be needed to implement a standard that hasn't been decided on yet.

A Senate judiciary committee began talks on this subject in December of 2007 under the guidance of Senator Whitehouse.[37] If the DEA standards are agreed on, the ability to e-prescribe controlled substances will diffuse through the e-prescribing software vendors, passing through development and integration teams, into upgrades and new products, and on to the final users. That takes time. If industry conventions are agreed on, users might see e-prescribing of controlled substances much sooner.

Question: How easy is it for someone to fraudulently use the e-prescribing application for noncontrolled substances?

Answer: It's a lot harder than stealing a prescription pad. Medical staff and personnel associated with a physician's office or hospital commit most diversion and prescription abuse. The portability of paper prescriptions make them easy targets, especially prescription pads that aren't serially numbered and tracked. E-prescribing has many security features that make unauthorized prescribing very difficult.

Question: Does e-prescribing violate HIPAA?

Answer: No. E-prescribing is allowed under HIPAA's "treatment, payment, and operations" exemption, but all the requirements of HIPAA electronic security apply.[25] Staff may need additional training on HIPAA requirements for electronic records such as keeping passwords safe, keeping monitors locked or turned off when not in use, and using fax cover sheets. Additional patient consent may be required. The issue becomes particularly complicated when higher level integration is desired, such as when discussing access privileges to information an HIE manages. (A full discussion of HIPAA requirements, including business associate agreements, patient consent, and security is beyond the scope of this book; others, such as Hale and Greenberg and colleagues[26] have covered this area well.[38] Another excellent resource for HIPAA questions is www.hhs.gov/ocr/hipaa/.)

Question about Safety

Question: Is e-prescribing safer than paper prescriptions?

Answer: Yes, but it doesn't eliminate errors.[21,39,40] The advent of electronic prescribing and prevalence of computerized physician order entry systems in hospitals resolved many safety concerns related to illegible orders[2,11,41] and created new types of errors in the process.[1,16,42–44] Reading the electronic prescription is no longer an issue, although understanding it can be. The pharmacist might wonder whether the prescriber really wanted the acetaminophen to be given intranasally. An order written for hydroxyzine 25 mg four times daily for blood pressure is ambiguous. The intended drug could be hydralazine, or the indication could be for itching instead of blood pressure.

The legibility hole in the dike of medication safety is plugged, though more solutions are needed to restore integrity to our medication use systems.[12,45] Electronic prescribing applications are a quantum leap forward in patient safety,[14] yet a new kind of awareness is needed by the clinician when using these applications to avoid different kinds of errors. See also Chapter 9.

Pharmacist Perspective

Medication safety is an important feature of e-prescribing that does nothing to lessen the pharmacist's role as a safety sentinel for the patient.[46] In fact, collaboration between prescribers and pharmacists is an effective way to harness e-prescribing to drive patient safety.[47] The challenge for the pharmacist is becoming attuned to the new ways that errors may sneak through on electronic prescriptions. See also Chapter 9.

Questions about Time and Efficiency

Question: Will e-prescribing save time?

Answer: Whether time is saved depends on who is asking the question. The improved legibility may reduce the number of pharmacy call-backs.[14,48] E-prescribing may reduce the amount of time prescription renewals take, and renewals drive most of the prescription volume in a primary care office. As a result, nonphysician staff heavily involved in prescription renewals may save the most time.[13] The choice of e-prescribing application, presence of **clinical decision support (CDS)**, experience with e-prescribing, and use of e-prescription–enabled pharmacies influence the actual time savings experienced.[49] For many prescribers, writing an e-prescription takes about as much time as a paper prescription.[18,49]

E-prescribing has many safety-rich features that make it easier for the prescriber and staff to provide quality care to patients, such as just-in-time drug information, patient medication lists, labels for drug samples, patient drug information, and formulary preferences. Without e-prescribing, these features and services would take considerably more time to provide.

(Rx) Pharmacist Perspective

E-prescriptions reduce the number of illegible faxes and clogged interactive voice systems. Fewer calls to insurance companies for formulary changes are needed and patient satisfaction usually increases. Renewal requests for existing prescriptions save the most time for the pharmacist.[9] From a safety perspective, voice messages and written prescriptions are inferior to properly implemented e-prescribing. By way of illustration, imagine a string of prescriptions on the pharmacy voice mail in a thick accent rattling off quinine, quinidine, rabeprazole, omeprazole, tizanidine, nizatidine, or any number of other sound-alike drugs.[41]

Question: Will e-prescribing take me away from my patients?

Answer: No. The amount of time spent with or away from the patient depends on how e-prescribing is used. One configuration and workflow choice creates a barrier between the prescriber and the patient. Another configuration and choice engages both prescriber and patient in productive discussion. If barriers are present, they represent unresolved challenges in the office more than challenges with the technology itself. See also Chapter 11.

Question: How much time for e-prescribing training is needed?

Answer: Allow a total of 4 hours training and 4 hours practice for each staff member. Training length will vary by person and by the e-prescribing functions for which that person is responsible. Just as there are people with extensive computer and clinical experience who can learn the basics within an hour, there are others who think closing a window keeps the warm air in, a mouse is a furry rodent, and a hard drive is more than 300 yards on a golf course. Medical office staff represent the spectrum of competence. Take the basic skills that individuals bring, mix it with the variety of roles each person can play, add a dash of strong personalities and you begin to get a picture of the training challenges ahead. See also Chapter 10.

Pharmacist Perspective

Training requirements for e-prescribing in the pharmacy is much the same as the requirements for an upgrade to the pharmacy software. Most features are straightforward with the way prescriptions are received and renewal requests are sent. Key safety areas to assess when reviewing an e-prescription are discussed in Chapter 9. Indeed, it is these areas of patient safety that should receive attention in pharmacy e-prescribing training. Failure to involve all pharmacy personnel may result in an e-prescription that languishes unfilled. The prescriber may then feel justified in his or her assessment that pharmacies are not ready for e-prescriptions.[38] At worst, a patient's therapy could be delayed.

Question about Special Circumstances

Question: I work in a specialty, and I'm retiring soon. Do the e-prescribing benefits apply to me?
Answer: Yes. Patients benefit the most from e-prescribing. Drug interaction checks, formulary alerts, **medication history (Hx)**, and improved legibility all combine to substantially increase patient safety. See also Chapter 7. Whether engaged in a specialty or nearing retirement, anyone writing prescriptions should strongly consider the electronic alternative.

Conclusion

The exploration of these questions demonstrates that both prescribers and pharmacists are involved on different sides of the same technological learning curve. The issues are complex and stretch across many disciplines. Having an appreciation of the entirety of e-prescribing from the prescriber, nurse, office manager, and pharmacist roles is essential to developing a sensitivity to the safety issues involved. The remainder of the book expands on some of these questions and delves into new areas we haven't touched on yet.

E-Prescribing Infrastructure

 READING PRIORITY

Finding a common place to begin a discussion of electronic prescribing is difficult. E-prescribing engages multiple disciplines but shows a different face to each one. We need to look beyond the surface of e-prescribing to the foundations applicable to every user. Only then will we understand the boundaries of this useful tool and, with the boundaries in view, apply the tool in a way that provides efficient, safe patient care.

This chapter covers a brief history of e-prescribing, the laws that allow it, the infrastructure that supports it, and the standards that define it. Technology can introduce new communication options, but dialogue is needed between the disciplines to create interdisciplinary solutions. This chapter provides the foundation for that dialogue to take place.

Clinical Corner

A prescriber sends an e-prescription to a pharmacy and sees no drug interaction alert flags, yet the pharmacist calls back with a concern about a serious drug interaction. What happened?

(continues)

Clinical Corner *(continued)*

Answer: The prescriber's alert settings may not be sensitive enough to trap the drug interaction, or the medication history in the e-prescribing application may be incomplete.

E-Prescribing and Government

The federal government is friendly to electronic prescribing. In 2003, the Medicare Modernization Act required the creation of standards for the transmission of electronic prescriptions addressing eligibility and benefits information, the medication history, the act of prescribing, and the medication profile. This task fell to the National Committee on Vital Health and Human Statistics, which convened several meetings in 2004 to evaluate existing standards. The work from these pivotal meetings led to the adoption of e-prescribing's **foundation standards**; their final ruling took effect in January 2006. This represented the first set of **final standards** prior to the CMS testing of the **initial standards**.[50]

Important Note

The standards define the manner in which electronic prescriptions for Medicare D recipients must be sent; they do *not* require prescribers to e-prescribe. If a prescriber chooses to use e-prescribing, any prescriptions generated for a Medicare D covered drug for a Medicare D recipient must conform to the standards.[50] In 2007, CMS removed the exemption for computer-generated faxes (effective January 1, 2009), leaving the EDI transaction as the only option available for electronic prescriptions.[28]

There is a strong movement within the government recommending mandatory e-prescribing for Medicare D patients.[51] If successful, this movement will cement the importance of these standards directly in the daily work of each prescribing clinician.

With the foundation standards defined, CMS undertook a pilot study in 2006 to test proposed standards with less industry experience.[52] The results, released in January of 2007, demonstrated the standards for medication history exchange and formulary/benefit information were stable. Standards for **RxNorm**, electronic **prior authorization**, and structured patient instructions need more work before they can be adopted.[2] A second set of final standards proposed in November 2007 incorporated the experience of the CMS pilot: use of the **national provider identifier (NPI)**, medication history, and formulary/eligibility standards.[53] The full, final set of uniform standards is expected to take effect on April 1, 2009.

Long-Term Care Exemption

The current **NCPDP SCRIPT standard (SCRIPT)** does not meet the workflows and legal responsibilities of long-term care, and modifications to the standard are under way to accommodate these unique needs. Until then, long-term care has an exemption that reads:

> Entities transmitting prescriptions or **prescription-related information** where the prescriber is required by law to issue a prescription for a patient to a non-prescribing provider (such as a nursing facility) that in turn forwards the prescription to a **dispenser** are exempt from the requirement to use the NCPDP SCRIPT standard adopted by this section in transmitting such prescriptions or prescription-related information.[50, p.67594]

While e-prescribing was making headway at the federal level, individual state governments began passing legislation favorable to e-prescribing, though discussing the intricacies of each state's laws is beyond the scope of this book.

Working definitions of electronic prescribing, electronic transmission, and **electronic media** vary by state. The CMS definition of e-prescribing expands the concept of transferring prescription information in an EDI transaction to include prescription-related information required for clinical decision support. Also, the CMS definition of electronic media specifically excludes facsimile transmissions.[50] This book will use the CMS definition of e-prescribing throughout for the sake of clarity.

As of 2007, electronic prescriptions for controlled substances are not allowed, though the industry is working with the government on standards that will allow this in the future.[34,35,54]

E-prescribing vendors may not be aware of your state-specific needs. The presence of another medical office or pharmacy in the state using the vendor's application is not sufficient proof that the vendor meets all the legal requirements. Sometimes a vendor upgrades its application and functionality needed

Sampling State Regulations

Alabama regulations do not consider the electronic prescription a written prescription. In contrast, New York has regulations that govern the electronic transmission of prescription information and specifically address facsimile transmissions. Ohio has *electronic* added as a descriptor of communication for prescriptions without making specific distinctions between transmissions or written prescriptions.

Many boards of pharmacy provide links to laws and regulations or address e-prescribing on their web sites. Answers can frequently be found by searching the laws and regulations with the keyword *electronic*. A listing of state boards of pharmacy and their web sites can be found at www.edhayes.com/sbp-main.html.

 Pharmacist Perspective

The New York State Board of Pharmacy has an excellent summary for handling faxed prescriptions that is worth repeating here:[36]

> The best professional judgment of the pharmacist is the key to a safe and effective process. The steps used to verify phoned prescriptions may also be useful for faxed prescriptions. These steps may include:
>
> - Calling the prescriber's office to verify a prescription if the prescriber is not known to the pharmacist;
>
> - Accepting a phoned in prescription in lieu of the faxed or computer transmitted prescription;
>
> - Asking for proof of identity if the person picking up the prescription is not known to the pharmacist;
>
> - Asking prescribers in the area to use an identifier on the faxed prescription form that indicates recopying or retransmittal. Such marks are commonly used to indicate if that document has been copied from an original;
>
> - Ensuring that the prescribed drug, based on quantity, directions for use, etc., is consistent with the patient's medication profile;
>
> - Using other methods such as installing "Caller ID" on the phone line that is used to receive fax prescriptions; and

(continues)

Pharmacist Perspective *(continued)*

> • Considering whether the prescribed drug is one with an abuse potential or otherwise has "street value."
>
> Without special safeguards, e-mail transmissions do not independently assure the required confidentiality of patient records and do not, therefore, meet the definition of an electronically transmitted prescription in the new [New York State] rules and regulations. If a pharmacist has reason to question the authenticity of the electronically transmitted prescription, the pharmacist's professional judgment must prevail.
>
> The New York State Board of Pharmacy web site can be accessed at www.op.nysed.gov/pharmelectrans.htm.

to comply with the law is lost. It is the user's responsibility, not the vendor's, to ensure the tools used in clinical practice are in conformance with the law.

Strict States Force Forms

New York State law article 137, section 6810 (6)(a), places stringent requirements on the form of the prescription. Since e-prescribing also involves printing prescriptions, the vendor needs to produce a format that accommodates this law.

Infrastructure Companies

Electronic prescribing draws together information and resources from different sectors of health care and weaves it into a single application (see **Figure 2.1**). Companies such as SureScripts, **RxHub**, eRx Networks, and RelayHealth technologies deliver the infrastructure that supports e-prescribing with valuable information and services, including patient eligibility, health plan formularies, patient benefits and co-pays, medication history, and prescription routing.

The Information Sources

Insurers drive the information content for the infrastructure companies, according to their ability. Not every insurer is able to contribute information across every category of patient eligibility checking, medication histories,

Spotlight on RxHub

Pharmacy benefits managers (PBMs) provide services to the insurance industry as their descriptive name indicates. In 2001, three of the largest PBMs, Merck-Medco, Advance PCS, and Express Scripts formed the company RxHub. They intended to provide a means of linking physicians with pharmacies electronically for the purposes of sending electronic prescriptions. In addition to e-prescription routing, RxHub also supports electronic prescribing with patient eligibility checking, medication histories, insurance plan formularies, and patient benefit and co-pay information. The three PBMs, along with subsequent partners RxHub has since added, cover an impressive number of lives, and their associated patient health information represents a valuable national information resource.[55]

insurance plan formularies, and patient benefit and co-pay information. For example, one insurer may be able to provide information on formularies alone while another can provide information in all four categories. The extent of the insurer's ability to provide content directly affects the clinician using e-prescribing.

Variability in information available from different insurers can result in apparent inconsistencies within the e-prescribing application. Formulary status without co-pay information may be available for one plan while a different plan includes both. It's not a fault of the e-prescribing program or the **interface** with the infrastructure provider; it's a result of the quality of the data available. Insurers are actively working to improve the quality and breadth of information provided with the result that far less variability will be experienced in the future.

Formulary Information

Insurance plans use formularies to control drug costs and pass the effects of those choices to prescribers, support staff, pharmacists, and patients. In the current environment, a prescriber writing a prescription on paper has little or no immediate access to the formulary. The consequences can be severe—the patient may not be able to afford the prescription. If they can afford the prescription, they may not take it as ordered, hoping to make the medication last as long as possible.

Insurers provide formulary information at the point of prescribing so that prescribers have the information available to choose a cost-effective alternative, if warranted. In fact, the

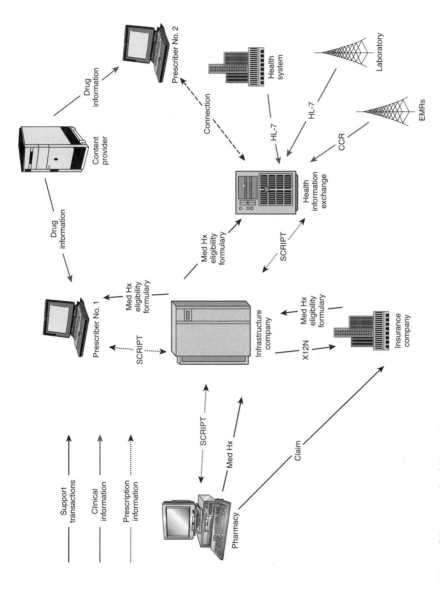

FIGURE 2.1 E-Prescribing Standards in Action

insurer often supplies a list of alternative medications in addition to the selected drug's formulary status. Insurers generally update their formulary information with infrastructure providers quarterly, though e-prescribing applications will typically check for formulary changes hourly, daily, or weekly.

Troubleshooting Tip

If you feel your formulary information is inaccurate, contact your e-prescribing application vendor. Something may be interfering with this regular formulary check.

In the e-prescribing application, the prescriber can see the formulary status of a selected medication for a patient based on the associated insurance.[56] Many e-prescribing applications also indicate whether the selected medication requires prior authorization, if identified as such by the insurer. Patients who can afford their medications are more adherent and enjoy better health, creating a win-win situation for everyone through a general reduction in medical expenses.

Formulary information is useful but may not display for every patient, potentially confusing the clinician. Consider the criteria needed to support the best-case scenario:

- The patient has a prescription benefit through an insurance plan that supplies formulary information to an infrastructure provider.

- The patient's prescription benefit is associated with the patient within the e-prescribing application.

The benefit of formulary information is lost if either of these conditions is missing. Some possible reasons include:

- The insurer is technologically unable to provide this level of information.

- The insurer does not have a relationship with an infrastructure provider.

- The e-prescribing application does not support identification of the pharmacy benefit provider.

- The office staff did not enter or correctly identify the patient's pharmacy benefit provider. For applications that automatically retrieve pharmacy benefit information, the patient information necessary for successful retrieval is missing or incomplete.

> **Formulary Fundamentals**
>
> Most three-tiered formularies consist of generic drugs in the first tier, followed by preferred brands in the second tier, followed by nonpreferred brands in the third tier. The patient's co-pay usually increases as the tier increases. The prescriber selecting a medication identified as third tier understands the patient usually incurs a greater expense as a result.

Eligibility

Eligibility information provided by insurers answers the question: *Does the patient have active prescription benefits or not?* When implemented in e-prescribing applications, eligibility checking may also look up the patient's insurance information using unique patient identifiers such as first name, last name, date of birth, gender, and zip code. When the insurance information is automatically populated, manual entry steps are saved. ✒

Clinically, the patient's status with the insurance has a direct effect on medication choices. If the patient is no longer active in the plan, previous formulary restrictions no longer apply. In the absence of any prescription coverage, the actual cost of the drug becomes the driving financial concern.

Benefits and Co-Pays

In 2008, few companies have the technological ability to provide patient co-pays and benefits information. When provided, the co-pay information drives the display of the patient's share in dollars and cents or, depending on the plan, as a percentage of drug cost. This allows the clinician to evaluate a selected medication's financial impact on the patient.

This co-pay information needs to be distinguished from pricing information that may be supplied by a product company such as First Databank, Multum, or Medispan. It is the vendor's responsibility to ensure the information is displayed in a way that clearly communicates to the prescriber the difference between co-pay and pricing if both are displayed. This is critically important in an environment where co-pay and pricing are inconsistently displayed as a result of limited data from information sources. As a clinician, understanding the difference between a display of the patient's co-pay and the average wholesale price of a drug is absolutely needed to make good decisions for the patient's therapy.

Medication Histories

What medications is a patient taking? Good clinical decisions depend on the answer to this question. The ideal patient medication history contains information about current and past medications including dietary supplements and over-the-counter (OTC) medications. The e-prescribing application adds the medication history to the **patient's profile**, allowing the prescriber to check drug interactions and view prescriptions written by others—an important safety feature.[57,58] Unfortunately we do not have a complete medication history solution, though the available histories are a giant leap forward.

When a patient with prescription coverage purchases a drug in a pharmacy, a claim is sent to the insurer for payment. The pharmacy computer has a record of dispensing for the medication. The insurer has a record of payment for the medication. Infrastructure providers mine this trail of information to deliver a medication history to the e-prescribing application.

Different Approaches, Similar Results

RxHub uses a federated model to retrieve the information. Like a giant switchboard operator, the request for medication history arrives from the e-prescribing application and is redirected to the appropriate insurer's data. The history is available across the nation.

SureScripts uses both a regionalized central data repository (CDR) to hold dispensing data from participating pharmacies and a federated model, depending on the needs of the information source. In the CDR model, the request for medication history from the e-prescribing application is matched to the patient's information in the central repository. The history is available for the supported regions and continues to expand as SureScripts adds resources.

An accurate medication history allows a provider to assess:

- Drug interactions—Is the patient taking medications that interact with other drugs, allergies, or diseases?

- Therapy appropriateness—Are there gaps in the current therapy? Are there therapies that should be stopped?

- Patient adherence challenges—Does the patient appear to be filling the medications appropriately?

- Duplications—Has another prescriber written for a similar medication? Is the patient still refilling an old medication?

Pharmacies and insurance claims are important sources of medication history information. The infrastructure providers are working hard to increase their ability to provide medication histories, but the clinician should be aware of their limitations, which include the following situations:

- The history may be incomplete. The information is retrospective in nature, reflecting a prescription that was paid for by the insurer. It does not capture prescriptions that have not been filled. Medications paid for with cash and not processed through an insurer will not appear in the claims database. Medications covered by insurers such as the Veteran's Administration (VA), Medicaid, or state insurance plans may not have a relationship with the infrastructure provider, and as such, will not contribute to the medication history. OTC medications purchased by the patient are not reflected in the history, nor are samples given to the patient. In fact, entire therapies may be sampled for months and never appear in the insurer's database.

  Likewise, the pharmacy dispense history may not represent all pharmacies. Prescriptions filled at nonparticipating pharmacies do not contribute medication history data. Pharmacy dispense data cannot account for sampled medications or medications dispensed in a medical office or clinic. OTC medications are not usually captured, although that may change in the future.

- The history doesn't indicate whether the patient picked the medication up at the pharmacy or used it, only that a claim was processed for it. As frequently happens in pharmacies, the claim may be submitted and reversed at a later date when the patient fails to pick up the order. This creates a small window of time in which the medication may appear active when it is actually on the pharmacy shelf waiting for the patient.

- The history does not reflect medication discontinuations or identify changes to the therapy. Any inferences based on claims data are assumptions. For example, determining if an order for lisinopril was changed to valsartan as opposed to intentionally adding valsartan to lisinopril is very difficult.

Despite these limitations, the value of the medication history is clear. In fact, combining pharmacy and insurer medication history data helps to

---

Helping Hands

Infrastructure providers contribute their resources to ICERx, an organization dedicated to bringing prescription information to healthcare professionals in the event of a disaster such as Hurricane Katrina. The ICERx web site can be accessed at www.icerx.org.

Pharmacist Perspective

Sometimes processing a patient's prescription through the insurer offers no financial benefit to the patient, especially in cases where the actual cost of the drug is less than the co-pay. Some pharmacists may avoid the additional work of sending the prescription to the insurer and simply charge the patient the cash price. ⊕ **It is important to realize that choosing not to process a prescription through a patient's insurer has a negative effect on medication histories.**

Communicating a patient's current insurer to the prescriber when a new prescription is needed, as in the case for prior authorizations and renewals, is a good practice. Medical offices record a patient's medical coverage, but tracking prescription benefit information is still new to them. An insurance company may have plans that provide pharmacy benefits through different PBMs. Giving the provider the information about the entity responsible for prescription coverage helps to keep the provider's records accurate and facilitates resolution of the issue at hand.

Spotlight on SureScripts

The National Association of Chain Drug Stores (NACDS) and the National Community Pharmacists Association (NCPA) jointly created SureScripts in 2001. The combined membership of these two national organizations encompasses the majority of our nation's pharmacies. SureScripts created the Pharmacy Health Information Exchange to act as a clearinghouse for e-prescriptions, providing a medium through which information can travel from prescriber to pharmacy and back again. In addition to the service of routing and handling e-prescriptions, SureScripts provides a mechanism for prescriber verification, maintains a database of pharmacies capable of receiving e-prescriptions, and certifies both pharmacy and prescriber applications for basic e-prescribing functions. In 2007, SureScripts added the services of providing medication history, formulary, and eligibility checking.[48]

minimize gaps since prescriptions filled through the pharmacy application are captured regardless of payer.

E-Prescribing Certification

SureScripts provides the certification of software for certain e-prescribing functions. **The National Council for Prescription Drug Programs (NCPDP)** created a standard for transmitting prescription information called

> **℞ Pharmacist Perspective**
>
> Never before have community pharmacy medication profiles played such a prominent role in the prescriptive process. Because the SureScripts medication history information relies on this pharmacy information, it is imperative to ensure the pharmacy's patient profile is as complete as possible. Medications dispensed by other pharmacies and OTC medications need to be included, though not all pharmacy applications support the ability to add these details.
> ⊕ **An accurate profile enhances the patient's safety every time a prescriber uses a pharmacy-based history to write an e-prescription for him or her.**

SCRIPT. SureScripts ensures this standard is applied correctly and that information travels between pharmacists and prescribers as intended. Basic certification verifies that new e-prescriptions travel from prescriber to pharmacist and requests for prescription renewals travel from pharmacist to prescriber.[59]

> **Tricky Terminology**
>
> It is important to underscore the definitions for *refill* and *renewal*. Many healthcare settings use these terms interchangeably, which leads to confusion in the context of e-prescribing. A prescription contains refills. One prescription can be refilled multiple times. When a prescription is expired or has no refills left, it is renewed. A renewal is the generation of a new prescription based on a previous prescription.

Optional certification is available for the SCRIPT transactions that allow a prescription to be cancelled (prescriber to pharmacist communication) or changed (pharmacist to prescriber communication).

E-Prescription Routing

The infrastructure companies provide a common interface for the delivery of electronic prescriptions. Instead of creating a separate interface for every pharmacy application in use, an e-prescribing vendor only needs to manage an interface with the infrastructure companies, which in turn communicate with the pharmacy applications.

Prescriptions may be sent through the infrastructure companies as an EDI or fax transaction. A successful EDI transaction requires the presence of compatible applications in both the prescriber's office and pharmacy. If the pharmacy or medical office lacks the ability to receive an EDI transaction, the information is converted into a computer-to-fax transmission. In the majority of situations, this occurs automatically or semiautomatically and is largely transparent to the clinician.

The clinician should be aware of the patient safety implications this represents. E-prescribing provides the greatest benefits when prescriptions are sent as an EDI transaction.

A computer-to-fax transmission still needs to be entered into the pharmacy dispensing application, opening up the potential for transcription error.

Also, the application sending the transaction as a fax may not conform to the e-prescribing standards with the result that some fields required by the standard, including drug name, dose, route, and patient information, may be incomplete or incorrect.

The infrastructure companies have security precautions to discourage prescriptions from unlicensed persons from traveling through the network, which complement the e-prescribing application's registration process. Every effort is made to verify the legitimacy of prescribers sending prescriptions through the network utilizing a combination of license and identity verification. As a result, prescribers not recognized as such by the infrastructure companies are unable to utilize prescription routing services regardless of their settings in the e-prescribing application.

Spotlight on eRx Network

The eRx Network began in 2001 as a new pharmacy transaction services company focused on providing the best value, service, and products to retail pharmacy. In March of 2005, eRx Network merged with Allwin Data, a leading provider of specialty pharmacy claims processing. The eRx Network provides billing services and data center solutions for pharmacists, long-term care facilities, pharmacy practice management vendors, and other healthcare professionals. The company now counts among its customers several major regional pharmacy chains, co-op groups, nationwide franchise groups, software vendors, and a sizeable base of independent pharmacies.

Through eRx Network, pharmacies have a choice in e-prescribing connectivity, similar to choosing a telephone long-distance carrier. For pharmacies that have unique needs such as long-term care or home health care, or for pharmacies with older applications, eRx Network can provide a solution that works with the existing infrastructure, connecting to SureScripts when needed or providing a direct connection to the physician's application.[60]

Spotlight on RelayHealth

In January of 2007, McKesson acquired Per Se technologies and leveraged the resources into a new business called RelayHealth. The goal of the new Relay-Health business is to improve how physicians, hospitals, pharmacies, payers, and patients share information, interact, and collaborate to improve the quality of care. To support quality care improvements and reduced administrative costs across the healthcare industry, RelayHealth operates as a neutral partner in an open network environment, offering connectivity and interoperability among all organizations, systems, and solutions,[61,62] including:

- Pharmacy transaction processing

- Financial transaction processing for payers and providers

- Physician–patient connectivity and care management tools and services that connect physicians with their patients, other physicians, providers, pharmacies, and payers

Infrastructure Summary

Clinical Corner

A new patient presents to his primary care provider (PCP) and states his heart medication made him feel tired for the last few months. The PCP views the patient's medication history but doesn't see any heart medications, though every other medication the patient reports is present. However, the patient's records show that his wife takes heart medication. Did someone inadvertently write the wrong name on the prescription? Did the patient mistakenly take his wife's medication? Is there another explanation?

The PCP understands there may be gaps in the medication history and inquires about other providers, specifically the VA. In fact, the patient does receive the prescription through the VA, and reports his other medications are more cost-effective through his health insurance. The information is updated in the e-prescribing application and the prescriber works with the VA to find the best therapy for the patient.

Insurers and pharmacies provide content to e-prescribing users through infrastructure providers. Understanding the information's source, the types of information provided, and the criteria needed for the information to display help the user troubleshoot problems and proactively avoid errors.

Content Providers

Most e-prescribing applications provide a searchable database of drug names, formulations, and patient instructions. The widespread integration of these databases into many e-prescribing applications serves to standardize the user's experience, which is helpful from a safety perspective. Drug information databases are usually licensed from content providers such as Medispan, First Data Bank, Epocrates, Multum, and others. These companies may also supply patient drug monographs, drug pricing, and drug interaction information to drive the application's clinical decision support. For the e-prescribing vendor, these databases greatly speed up application development and help them bring their product to market sooner.

The gains in application development are offset by a loss in flexibility for clinician-requested enhancements.[63,64] Changes in the e-prescribing application to the drug search logic, patient instructions, and interaction alerts now involve the product company in addition to the e-prescribing vendor. This may delay the needed change or prevent it from going through at all.

A survey of different e-prescribing applications will demonstrate a variety of interfaces and displays. Though the information supplied by the product company is relatively consistent, the manner in which the information is displayed depends on the e-prescribing application vendor. A good implementation enhances patient safety while a poor implementation detracts from it. The interaction of product companies and e-prescribing vendors affect nearly every part of e-prescribing, and the safety implications are discussed throughout the book.

Pharmacist Perspective

The way drugs are presented to the prescribers contributes greatly to the potential for error. A poor e-prescribing application may send extraneous abbreviations such as *TBCH* for chewable tablet. When in doubt, clarify with the prescriber.

Other good practices:

- Keep a log of strange abbreviations sent by e-prescribing applications for the benefit of other pharmacy staff.
- Ask the patient if he or she received and understood drug information from the prescriber.

(continues)

Pharmacist Perspective *(continued)*

- Never assume a prescriber saw an interaction unless he or she specifically documented it on the e-prescription. Alert fatigue is responsible for many ignored warnings.[65–67] Some prescribers turn off alerts entirely.

The Standards

Refining RxNorm

RxNorm is a publicly available drug nomenclature database produced by the National Library of Medicine that began as a project in 2001.[68] RxNorm is still maturing as a standard, as the CMS pilot demonstrated. Even so, some newer e-prescribing applications use RxNorm as their database to drive the display of drug choices during prescription writing. The older e-prescribing applications with a history stretching back to the 1990s and continuing into the early 2000s usually have a relationship with a product company to provide their medication information.

NCPDP SCRIPT

The National Council for Prescription Drug Programs developed a standard for electronically communicating prescription information called SCRIPT. In practice, prescription information is packaged into the SCRIPT standard when traveling between the pharmacy and the prescriber computers.

 SureScripts provides certifications for applications that handle e-prescriptions to ensure this standard is implemented appropriately and works as intended. Basic certification includes NEWRX and REFREQ, while **RXCHG** and CANRX are optional certifications.

Certification verifies the information received is the same as the information sent. The vendor is responsible for the implementation or display of the standards within the application.

This variability among vendors contributes to the potential for error in e-prescribing applications. Table 2.1 lists the segments of information common to NCPDP transactions.

NEWRX (Basic)

The NEWRX transaction is used to send a new prescription from the prescriber to the pharmacy. Regardless of whether the prescription is actually new or a new copy of an existing prescription, this is the transaction type used.

TABLE 2.1 Common Segments Used in NCPDP SCRIPT[71]

Segment	Purpose
PVD	Provider information
PTT	Patient information
DRU	Drug information
OBS	Observation; included if needed
COO	Coordination of benefits—may contain information on the patient's prescription program. Included if needed.

Source: Adapted from NCPDP. Prescriber/Pharmacist Interface SCRIPT Standard. Implementation Guide, Version 60: National Council for Prescription Drug Programs; 2004.

REFREQ (Basic)

The refill request transaction is unfortunately named since it refers to a request for renewal. When an existing prescription in a pharmacy application has expired and authorization is needed to continue the therapy, the REFREQ is used. As such, the communication travels from the pharmacy's computer to the prescriber's.

RXCHG (Optional)

The prescription change request transaction allows a pharmacist to request a change to a new prescription. Perhaps a lower cost generic agent or therapeutic alternative is needed. Whatever the reason, the prescriber's original prescription can be sent back with pharmacist-suggested changes.

CANRX (Optional)

The cancel prescription transaction communicates discontinuation of a therapy to the pharmacy. In today's environment, the pharmacy is rarely informed when a therapy has been changed or discontinued. The CANRX function is critical when the prescriber, pharmacist, nurse, or other professional administering the medication all need to understand which orders are active and which have been stopped.

HL-7 and CCR

Health Level 7 (HL-7) is a standard typically used in the hospital setting to convey clinically relevant patient information.[69] Computerized physician order entry (CPOE) systems are the hospital's equivalent of e-prescribing, and most of these systems use the HL-7 standard.

What happens when a hospital clinic wants to send a prescription to a community pharmacy? Different solutions are used to accomplish the task and usually involve changes to the CPOE application and clinic workflow. Though HL-7 is a standard, its implementation can vary greatly between applications. NCPDP and HL-7 standards are under examination by the industry to create a clear transition between the two.[70] In the future, hospital systems and community systems will work together more smoothly.

The continuity of care record (CCR) is an emerging standard whose base resides in **electronic health records (EHR)** and EMR. The CCR contains clinically relevant patient and insurance information, including drug information.[38] How does information in the EHR make its way into an e-prescribing application or a pharmacy? This higher level of integration is of special interest to the RHIOs and creators of HIEs. As the technology matures, the development of interfaces between the standards continues.

Eligibility Standard X12N

The **X12N 270/271** standard is utilized when checking a patient's eligibility status with an insurer through an infrastructure company. As an added convenience to the prescriber, the eligibility transaction may also identify the correct pharmacy benefits provider. Though the standard is widely used, its value is diminished by technology limitations across insurers that prevent them from fully interacting with the infrastructure companies. Convergence of technology and information sources will enhance future utility. This standard may be used, along with SCRIPT and HL-7, to enable electronic prior authorizations in the future.

Conclusion

Understanding that different standards exist for different functions and what those standards do lays the foundation for safely using the technology. For example, a prescriber who needs to communicate discontinuation orders to the pharmacy understands the CANRX transaction is optional and contacts the vendor to add that functionality. The industry is surging forward on multiple fronts with the result that the challenges identified in this chapter will shrink over the coming years.

PART II

The Tools

Chapter 3

E-Rx Anatomy– Assistant Functions

READING PRIORITY

Prescribers . . . . Required
Nurses/medical assistants . . . . Required
Office managers . . . . Suggested
Pharmacists . . . . Suggested
E-Rx application designers . . . . Required

Introduction

In February of 2007, Allscripts released eRx NOW, a web-based e-prescribing application freely available to prescribers.[3] The next three chapters dissect the functions of a typical e-prescribing application to illustrate the relevant safety topics, and the eRx NOW application is used as a visual example when screen shots are needed. The functions and features implemented in eRx NOW are similar to those found in other e-prescribing applications, and the easy access that readers have to this tool make it useful for illustration purposes; the author neither promotes nor maligns the eRx NOW product. Readers can get an overview of the current application through the tutorials at http://erxnow.allscripts.com.

---

eRx Now Notes

The web-based nature of the eRx NOW application lends itself to a dynamic and constantly evolving improvement process. The screen shots used for demonstration purposes may not reflect the current application. In recognition

(continues)

> **eRx Now Notes (continued)**
>
> of this, the screen shots provided are meant to provide examples of general e-prescribing features common to most applications or illustrative of a concept expressed in the text as opposed to features or challenges unique to eRx NOW.

Every e-prescribing application, whether it is part of an EMR or stand-alone solution, needs to provide a supportive environment for the user to manage prescriptions, such as intuitive navigation, logical data management, and simple data manipulation. Patient information and medication orders are entered, edited, and deleted. Once the information is there, the application sends it, relates it to other information, rearranges it, organizes it, combines it, and divides it.

From this understanding of e-prescribing's basic functions, we'll explore enhanced functions important for their potential benefit to safety. Some of these enhanced functions are present in e-prescribing applications other than eRx NOW, while others are not present in any application. The purpose in discussing them is threefold: to give readers a deeper understanding of the functions encountered by the assistant using e-prescribing, to give specific functions to submit as enhancement requests with the current vendor (see also Chapter 8—just because these functions didn't exist in 2007 doesn't mean they won't be available in 2009), and to raise an overall awareness of the way patient safety is affected by current and future functions.[71]

Just-In-Time Information

A supportive environment provides information in a timely and relevant fashion, and nearly every e-prescribing application employs just-in-time information (JITI) in one fashion or another. Each application will employ its own conventions, giving JITI a unique appearance according to the application.

Let's take a moment to examine the way eRx NOW handles JITI in the areas of formulary status, formulary alternatives, clinical drug alerts, context-sensitive interface changes, and an embedded Google search option.

During the prescribing process, icons representing the formulary status of the medication communicate the relative cost to the patient and the insurer. If the patient's drug coverage is changed within the application, the formulary status of each medication changes as well. In addition, the formulary alternatives displayed during the prescribing process reflect the change in insurance.

A subtle example of JITI is the way that interface elements are enabled or disabled depending on the active screen element. This workflow information is a further refinement of forcing functions. For example, a prescription cannot be generated unless a patient is selected. The option to create a prescription is not selectable unless the previous condition exists (having a patient selected).

The embedded Google search is one step removed from true JITI. Its presence allows rapid access to the information on the internet but still requires several user manipulations to get there.

Efficient use of existing information also enhances patient safety. During prescribing, selection of a drug or order will automatically populate the search field, reducing the number of steps to retrieve information and decreasing the potential for miskeyed search terms.

Just as formulary alternatives are displayed when a medication is selected, JITI displays the CDS alerts (see Chapter 7 for examples). **This preview, as with formulary icons, enables the prescriber to alter the choice of drug before going through the extra steps of writing out the patient instructions, quantity dispensed, days supplied, and refills.**

JITI should be applied in areas outside the medication prescribing process.[72,73] A hint window that reveals information when the cursor hovers over a data element is one example. Imagine patient searching where a thumbnail of patient-specific information is displayed before selection. Imagine renewing a medication and being able to see a display of the last fill dates; or an indication of overdue, renewal too soon, or on-time status; or previous order comments. Imagine the administrator resetting a user's password and seeing the number of times the user has been locked out and when. Maybe retraining is needed. To reach its full potential, JITI should be joined with the CDS functions suggested in Chapter 7. Saturating JITI into all aspects of the e-prescribing application enhances efficiency and accessibility for users, which translates into enhanced safety for patients.

Patient Demographics

Figure 3.1 shows the patient edit screen for eRx NOW. The application enables rapid demographic entry through a reverse look-up process. When the user enters the patient's phone number, at least four databases are searched to retrieve and populate some of the key fields, minimizing data entry.

The rapid acquisition of patient demographic information is crucial to the successful use of the application. A long manual entry process increases the likelihood the prescriber will use a paper prescription or incompletely enter information in an attempt to speed up the prescription writing process.[18]

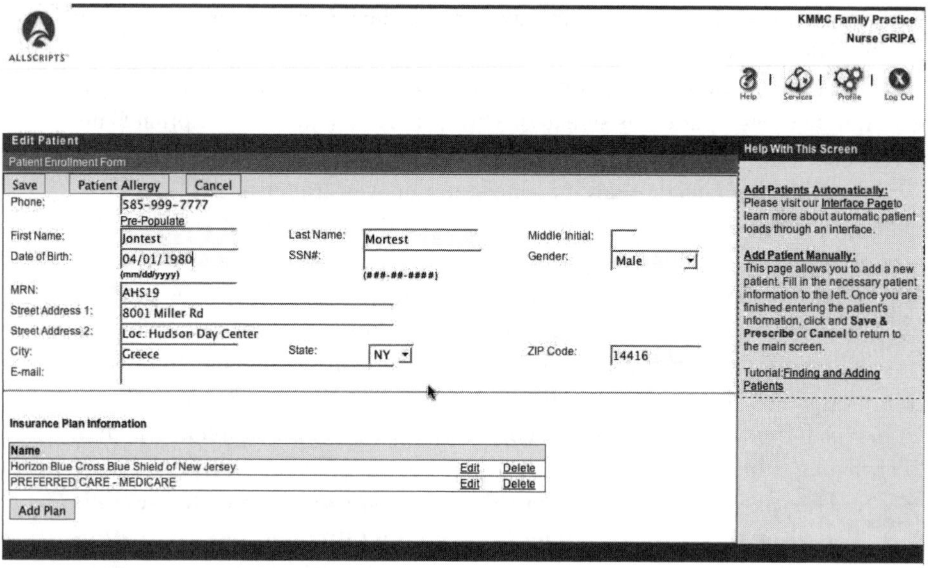

FIGURE 3.1 Patient Edit Screen
Source: Copyright 2007 Allscripts.

Automated solutions for acquiring patient demographics include interfaces between the e-prescribing system and another source of information such as an HIE or the practice management system. Even with automation, a solid manual-entry process is needed for situations that fall outside the activities

---

Patience with Patient Entry

The type of practice and workflow affects the need to enter patients manually. A specialist with a high volume of new patients may have a greater need for the manual entry function than a primary care provider with a low volume of new patients.

Existing workflow may also affect the need for manual entry. Even if an interface with a practice management system or EMR is used, manual patient registration in e-prescribing may be required if:

- A significant amount of time passes before patient data from the **practice management system (PMS)** updates the e-prescribing application
- The patient registration into the PMS or EMR system occurs after the patient's visit

Modifying the workflow to ensure patients are registered prior to the visit may avoid the need to use the manual registration function for e-prescribing.

covered by automation: on-call challenges, technical difficulties with the interfaces, and the unusual events that can never be described beforehand but only vaguely anticipated. The need to manually enter patients is unlikely to disappear.

Other actions are available from the patient demographics screen, such as the ability to add allergies and patient insurance information.

Note the ability to add allergies is also accessible from the patient header when the patient is initially selected—a good use of redundancy.

Patient Demographics Enhancements

We've discussed basic elements common to most e-prescribing applications. An enhanced, future application might include a family generator.

Internal medicine and family practice physicians care for families, not just individual patients. The family generator function could speed manual entry of families by keeping essential demographic information such as address and phone number constant for the next entry.

Creating relationships between patients adds another layer of protection and safety to the prescribing process. Imagine writing a prescription for a patient who shares the same name as his father. The relationship "Son of" as part of the demographic display or available in the contextual hint text helps to ensure the correct person is selected. Identifying these relationships is important in the larger, integrated environment. Understanding the social and familial relationships between patients has direct bearing on their health care and is valuable information for social workers, nurses, and other providers.

Understanding relationships is important for choosing medications as well. When a husband and wife are on the same medication but different doses, the chance for a **medication error** rises dramatically. Conversely, they may be on different drugs and similar doses—lovastatin 10 mg and atorvastatin 10 mg, for example. If the patient doesn't pay attention to the drug name, a misadministration may occur. Making relationships transparent to the prescriber may help to proactively avoid these situations.

In some cases, using the same medication within the family unit may promote nonadherence. What if the wife's drug is not a preferred formulary agent and costs three times as much? The wife might not take the medication at all, take it less frequently than prescribed to spread out the cost, or take her husband's medication (hopefully, it's the same dose).

Sometimes using the same drug is simply expedient. Sometimes the patient needs an explanation of the rationale for a different therapeutic agent used to treat the same condition in the same family. For example, why would amlodipine be used for the husband while isradipine is used for the wife? Perhaps the doses would be different and the purpose would be to avoid an administration error—which is reasonable but needs to be explained to the patient.

The ability to call up related medication profiles in the same house is one step closer to treating the family unit as a whole instead of each patient in isolation. When variances in patient administration do occur, the ability to view familial relationships and profiles may prove useful.

 Including more detailed contact information, which can drive address book functions such as e-mail, phone, fax, reports, and letters, extends the basic demographic functions of e-prescribing applications. Integrated patient address book functions may facilitate provider–patient communication such as sending patient drug information, providing an updated medication list, clarifying a medication's instructions, and more.

 Communication with the integrated healthcare community is enhanced with the addition of broadly applicable profile-level comments. Does the patient winter in Florida? Is there a language barrier? Is there a primary caregiver who should be contacted? This information is not contained in the medication order but is helpful to other healthcare providers involved in the patient's care.

Representing the next level of patient-oriented interaction, some vendors have begun development of patient interfaces for e-prescribing and healthcare applications.[74] It may be valuable to include patient-level comments on medication orders. Did the medication cause diarrhea or a rash? Is it too expensive? Did it successfully resolve the issue treated? This kind of feedback can be received and acted on in a way that wasn't previously possible.

Patient demographics are rich in healthcare-relevant information. E-prescribing applications should strive to make this important information more transparent to the users. Paying attention to details when making clinical decisions and automating the otherwise manual entry process as much as possible creates a safer process.

Problems, Diagnoses, and Procedures

Many e-prescribing applications, and especially those integrated with an EMR, have the capability of storing a patient's problems, diagnoses, and past procedures. This active problem list in a patient's profile contains a wealth of information for the prescriber and other healthcare professionals. The eRx NOW application offers two methods for entering diagnoses into the patient's profile: directly into the problem list and through the prescription-writing process.

When a prescriber selects a diagnosis and subsequently chooses a medication, the diagnosis is added to the patient's active problem list. The prescriber can either enter an **ICD-9** code or a fragment of text. The application then displays the closest matches for the diagnosis or procedure. One of the limitations of this useful function is that ICD-9 codes are not the most clinically recognizable description of a patient's diagnosis. This makes looking up a fairly straightforward condition such as breast cancer or hyperthyroidism very difficult.

Implementation Tip

In many applications driven by this ICD-9 list, the easier way to get the diagnoses into the system is to ask the person who does the office billing for the code, or have someone familiar with medical billing populate the active problem list.

Problems, Diagnoses, and Procedures Enhancements

Allowing the clinician to create a crosswalk from clinical terminology to the ICD-9 codes may bridge the gap between clinical and billing terminology. Some EMR systems already have this function and in the process support their e-prescribing component. With what code does hypertension correlate best? What about CHF? BPH? CAD? ASCVD? CKD? CVA? Medicine is filled with abbreviations for diagnoses and conditions that should be taken into account when creating a system to hold that information. Just as medications can be expressed by a brand name (sometimes multiple brands) and a generic name, diagnoses need a common reference list drawn from the way clinicians document health information.

Applications with support for an active problem list should provide a means of identifying which diagnoses are of greatest clinical concern. Is the diabetes well controlled while the heart failure requires frequent assessments and adjustments to the therapy? Or is the situation reversed, with the diabetes out of control and the heart failure mild and stable? Identifying the diagnosis with the greatest contribution to the patient's current health is particularly useful for healthcare providers seeing the patient for the first time.

Designer Details

A crude but potentially useful way to automate this level of priority is to evaluate the activity in the patient's profile related to the diagnoses. Diagnoses that have more medication changes and prescriptions attached to them rise higher in the priority list than diagnoses with little associated activity.

Another refinement needed in the integrated application **is a way to identify the primary manager of a condition.** Is the primary care physician writing orders for the patient's coronary artery disease or is the cardiologist managing it? Who is the primary manager of the patient's diabetes—the endocrinologist or the primary care provider? The ability to indicate a shared responsibility aids other healthcare providers who also access the patient's problem list. For example, this information may guide an emergency department physician to make a patient referral to the correct specialist for follow-up.

Allergies

Nearly every e-prescribing application accommodates patient allergies (see **Figure 3.2**). In eRx NOW, allergies are entered through the patient edit screen or directly from the patient header information that appears when the patient is selected. The allergy selection process resembles the medication selection process. Once the medication is selected, a reaction can be attached, or, if it is not found on the list, it can be entered as a free-text entry. Having reactions for allergies is important for the clinician to weigh the risks and benefits of drug therapy.[75] The reaction could be a rash, excessive sleepiness, or hives. The nature of the patient's reaction determines the subsequent course of action.

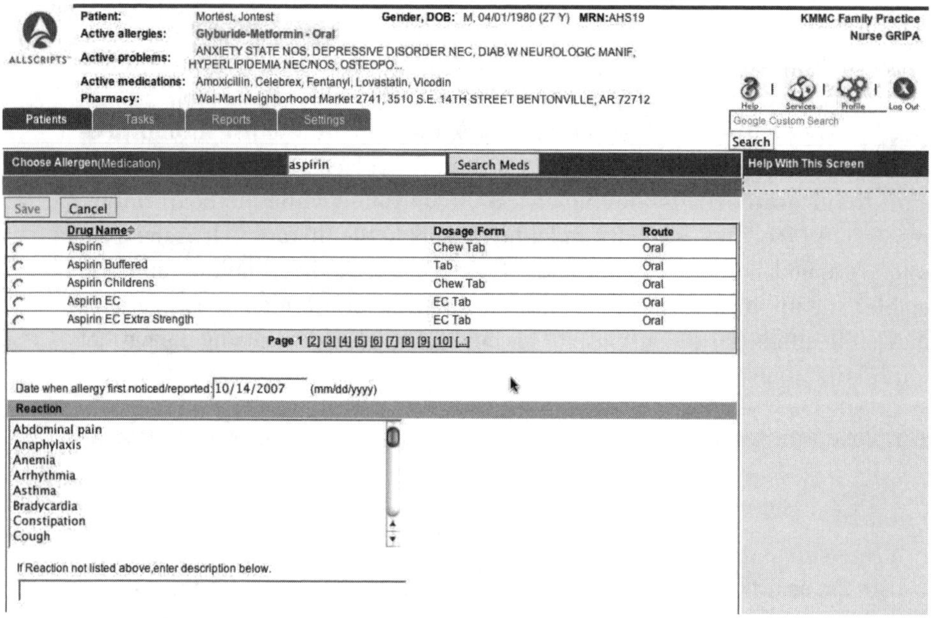

FIGURE 3.2 Choose Allergies
Source: Copyright 2007 Allscripts.

Allergies Enhancements

 Enhancing allergy selection is an important goal. Allergies are best represented by a medication's ingredients, not its formulation.[76]

The section for allergies can be enhanced by including several refinements. It is helpful to distinguish between a true allergic reaction, intolerance, and hypersensitivity. Allergies are immune-mediated in nature, intolerance indicates adverse effects were problematic, and hypersensitivity implies an extension of the drug's natural effect. The clinician's response to these categories is very different. A mild allergic reaction may require premedication with an antihistamine or steroid. An intolerance may be avoided using a drug with different pharmacologic properties, such as using a hydrophilic statin in place of a lipophilic statin for lowering cholesterol. A hypersensitivity response suggests lower doses may be needed for that medication and probably other drugs in the same pharmacological class. Designating the type of reaction is needed, though rarely supported, in the integrated application.

Many applications ignore the dual nature of allergies, which are antigenic class level and drug specific. True allergies are dealt with on a class level. For example, a patient has an allergy to penicillin—a class-level allergy in which cross-sensitivity is likely. Any drug related to penicillin is scrutinized for its potential to stimulate the same allergic-type reaction. When the immune system is involved, the stakes are higher.

Drug intolerances and hypersensitivities tend to be treated as drug-specific events. An upset stomach with ibuprofen is an example. While piroxicam may also cause similar gastric disagreement, there is a chance it will be better tolerated. The clinician is more disposed to trying another medication in the same drug family when an intolerance is present as opposed to an immunogenic allergy.

Abookire and comrades found that 65% of allergy alerts were not new alerts, but the same alert for a given patient that occurred each time the patient profile was accessed.[77] Selective suppression is needed for previously overridden allergy alerts that trigger when the medication is renewed. This could take the form of a passive, rather than active, display on medication renewal or a temporary suppression of the alert entirely.

When the prescriber identifies the patient as not having the allergy, the system should allow for editing or inactivating the allergy simultaneous with the alert. This facilitates the maintenance of current and accurate allergy data.

Most applications provide a way to select a specific medication and then apply the allergy across the drug class. What is needed is the choice to select a drug allergy as a specific drug or antigenic class. Selection of an individual drug without choosing to extend the allergy to the class, by default, could apply the allergy only to that individual drug.

As an example, **nonsteroidal anti-inflammatory drugs (NSAIDs)** could be selected in the allergy edit screen as a class of drugs that cause gastrointestinal bleeding for a patient recently on ibuprofen. Alternatively, ibuprofen could be entered as a drug-specific intolerance with the option of expanding the intolerance to include the entire class of NSAIDs.

Besides medications, the allergy section needs to accommodate environmental allergies. Patients with allergies to agents such as eggs, latex, milk, shellfish, iodine, and peanuts must also avoid certain medications. This is one place where formulation does matter, independent of the medication. For example, many vaccines are grown in chicken eggs and should be avoided in patients with a severe allergy to eggs.

As another application of JITI, medications triggering an allergy alert should be proactively identified during the order selection process of prescription writing similar to the way formulary icons are applied. The type of identification should be commensurate with the severity of the alert. For example, medications that will generate an allergy could be bolded, italicized, shaded, or have an icon attached.

In the eRx NOW application, a medication choice resulting in a potential allergy alert is shaded with an identifying mark, "DA" for drug allergy, appended to the choice. If the cursor is held over the medication, a tip appears that indicates the patient's reaction.

As with other clinical alerts, reverse functionality should be enabled. Reverse allergy checking scans the active drugs of a patient's profile when a new allergy is entered and provides appropriate alerts. Likewise, the clinician needs the opportunity to provide a reason for an allergy override.[76]

Lastly, to minimize alert fatigue, controls are needed to manage cross-sensitivity alerts.[75] An allergy to penicillin warrants an alert of potential cross-sensitivity when cephalexin is prescribed. An allergy to sulfa-based antibiotics should not trigger an alert when furosemide is prescribed.[78]

Designer Details

Applying cross-sensitivity alerts to class-level allergies while excluding drug-specific allergies provides cross-sensitivity controls in a crude fashion, but it assumes the application can differentiate between a class-level allergy and a drug-specific allergy.

Insurance

Identifying a PBM is essential to providing formulary information. The payer for a patient's medical claims is not always the same as the payer for the patient's drug benefit. Many e-prescribing applications provide eligibility checking as part of their functionality. This is a good feature in theory but needs time to mature. The utility of eligibility checking is reduced when local plans are not represented. For example, the major payers of health benefits such as the VA, state prescription plans such as EPIC (New York State drug coverage for the elderly), and Medicaid are frequently absent.

Filling the Gaps

Some state coverage plans require concomitant Medicare D coverage. This has two beneficial effects for e-prescribing users—the eligibility request will discover the Medicare D plan, and medication history can be obtained. Unfortunately, whether or not the patient is also receiving prescription benefits from the state plan is still not captured. Infrastructure companies are working to enroll new data providers to fill these information gaps for the future.

As the technology matures, more and more insurers will allow eligibility checking to occur. When this happens, proactive eligibility checking will be desirable in e-prescribing as a way of both increasing patient adherence and reducing telephone volume in the prescriber's office.

When a patient's insurance changes, medications once affordable under the previous insurance plan may become more expensive. In some cases, the patient may opt not to take the medication. In other cases, the patient makes phone calls to the medical office in an effort to find a less expensive alternative therapy. Changes to therapy in these conditions have a higher potential for error.

Having a proactive eligibility alert that runs when the profile is accessed, after the first of the year, or with any status change, is a powerful way for the prescriber to ensure the patient remains on the most cost-effective medications before the patient runs out of his current supply.

In eRx NOW, multiple insurers can be added to the patient's profile with the result that drugs are displayed with the most restrictive formulary tag. The ability to support multiple insurers is an important feature to look for in an e-prescribing application. Many patients, especially with the advent of Medicare Part D, have multiple pharmacy benefits that are additive with each other. This information is valuable when deciding on an expensive but necessary therapy—coverage by a secondary insurance may be the deciding factor.

Making Invisible Insurances Visible

Another feature to advocate for is the ability to free text an insurer that doesn't appear in the list. For example, noting the patient has benefits through the VA is important. If the e-prescribing application limits the choice of insurance to a predefined list that omits the VA, this information cannot be displayed. As a result, medications that are not on the VA's formulary may be ordered, resulting in additional expense for the patient or nonadherence. Even though the formulary status icons would not be visible with a free-texted insurance, the prescriber would at least be aware of the insurer and could alter the choice of prescriptions accordingly.

Medication Profile

The medication profile is the heart of the e-prescribing application, always present, supporting the prescriber and assistant alike. The medication profile drives the value of clinical alerts. The medication profile contains the active medication list. The medication profile is the source for prescriptions that need renewing and the record that organizes past medications.

The first challenge confronting any new user of an e-prescribing application is to populate the medication profile with the patient's existing medications. See Chapter 11. Both SureScripts and RxHub provide medication histories that make this task easier, though they are far from a complete solution. See Table 6.1. The formulation used to fill a prescription in a pharmacy may differ from the prescriber's notes. For example, if a prescriber chose a capsule formulation of ramipril and ordered half tablets, the pharmacy likely dispensed the tablet formulation of ramipril. Not all orders are represented in the prescriber's records, such as OTC medications and supplements. Orders derived from claims data and pharmacy data still need to undergo an internal reconciliation process within the office to ensure accuracy.

Figure 3.3 illustrates a basic view of the medication profile that includes the date the order was written, any associated problems or diagnoses, the order status, and the order itself. Advanced view options include the ability to sort by date or to filter the list by the prescription status to view active, inactive, or all prescriptions. Other applications have similar functions with varying degrees of flexibility in their displays.

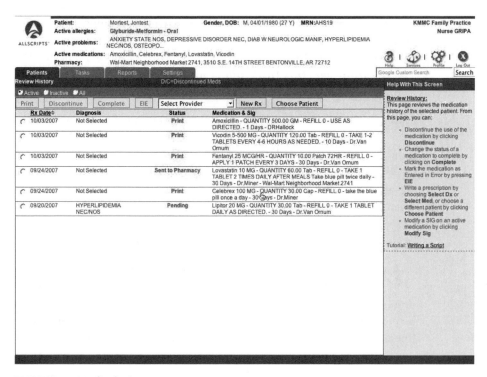

FIGURE 3.3 Medical History
Source: Copyright 2007 Allscripts.

Medication Profile Enhancements

The medication profile can be improved in many ways by extending the functions it currently performs. The medication profile serves as the single record for the prescriber to consult when deciding on the addition of a medication. It places that choice into the context of the patient's other medications. So what can assist the prescriber in making that decision?

Display Options

Providing an array of dynamic filters for the prescriber's or assistant's use is one way to organize medication orders in a way most relevant for patient care. Consider the utility of the following filters:

- *By Diagnosis:* This filter organizes a patient's medication list according to the primary diagnosis for which the medication was prescribed. In conjunction with the active problem list, this can highlight untreated indications.[71]

Many medications serve a dual purpose. For example, a beta blocker may be used for heart failure, coronary artery disease, high blood pressure, heart rate control, essential tremor, and migraine prophylaxis. A filter by therapies can provide insight into the best therapeutic option.

⊕ **In the integrated environment, where others have access to the medication list, this filter helps place the patient's therapies in the context of the patient's overall treatment plan.**

- ⊕ *By Discontinuation Reason:* Filtering the inactive medication list by discontinuation reason is a quick way to review previous therapies that have been tried. Perhaps a previous drug has been stopped due to its noncovered formulary status, but now the patient has a different insurance. Was a drug discontinued for intolerance such as mild diarrhea, or was it debilitating? Other healthcare providers using an integrated application to view patient data are able to make better decisions with this information at hand.

- ⊕ *By Patient Cost:* Displaying high-cost medications together in the profile assists in evaluating the overall financial burden a medication regimen represents. This view comes into its own when used to target expensive regimens for cost-effective alternatives. It's important to state the need for a patient-centric filter: the patient's co-pay should be used if an insurer is present, or the average wholesale price (AWP) should be used if no insurer is identified.

- ⊕ *By Level and Type of Alerts Currently in Effect:* Normally, alerts trigger during order entry and are not stored with the medication order. If the alert persisted with the order, this view could be used as a troubleshooting tool. In effect, each patient profile would have a record of currently interacting drugs, dose alerts, and allergy interactions available for review as needed. Sometimes a medication with an interaction is prescribed because the risk:benefit ratio favors the drug. When a patient presents with unusual side effects or new symptoms, sorting by the type of alerts attached to an order can help to narrow down the possible culprits to a list of likely suspects.

Evaluating Adherence

The medication history in eRx NOW displays the patient's active medication list as a moment frozen in time. For e-prescribing applications that have a chronological history, an evaluation of changes across the patient's therapy is possible. Embedded in each medication order is a history of renewals, helping to answer questions such as: Does the patient constantly request early renewals? Was the last prescription for diabetic medication over a year ago?

➕ The prescription history is a useful tool for the prescriber to assess patient adherence, particularly when displayed in a graphic form. Pharmacy fill data and claims data complement the e-prescribing application's history. A comparison of dates in a medication's fill history may uncover patterns of nonadherence that, depending on the pattern (see **Table 3.1**), point to a specific resolution.

TABLE 3.1 Nonadherence Patterns

Pattern	Likely Cause	Resolution
Refills are a multiple or fraction of the days supplied (Example: Quantity dispensed = 60, Days supply = 30, Patient refills every 60 days reflecting once-daily administration)	Incorrect administration	Verify administration instructions with the patient.
Refills are consistently 1 to 2 weeks late	Inconvenient regimen, financial concerns	Ask the patient about the gaps. Look for convenient, cost-effective therapies. Assess the need for memory-assist devices such as pill organizers.
Refills are separated by gaps of a month or more	Knowledge and understanding challenges	Assess the value the patient places on the therapy. Address gaps in knowledge and understanding.
Refills are consistent and become inconsistent	Changing insurance co-pays (Example: Medicare D patients)	Ask the patient if affording medications is more of a concern at one time of the year than another. Evaluate medications for cost-effectiveness and formulary adherence. Consider involving a social worker.
Refills are inconsistent and become consistent	Insurance deductible (Example: Medicaid spend down)	Ask the patient if affording medications is more of a concern at one time of the year than another. Evaluate medications for cost-effectiveness and formulary adherence. Consider involving a social worker.

Nonadherence should always be assessed before increasing the dose of a patient's medication for safety reasons. Failing to address nonadherence may result in unnecessary expense as treatments are labeled "failed" and more expensive options are tried. Patients who do become adherent at the increased dose may suffer adverse effects with the result that a treatment is labeled as "failed."

Designer Details

Providing a calendar with shaded days representing the days supplied by a prescription quickly communicates adherence. Any gaps between the amount of medication supplied and the time a new prescription was issued become immediately obvious.[13]

Selecting Medication Orders

From a prescription management perspective, the ability to select and perform actions on multiple orders within the medication profile is very useful. The patient might have just transferred to hospice care, requiring discontinuation of all the active prescriptions. A provider assuming care for a new patient would need to rewrite all the active prescriptions. Batch selection allows the discontinuation or renewal of many orders at once. The patient might be going to a new pharmacy. The user could send the whole batch to the pharmacy, printer, or the assistant at one time. This increases safety by greatly reducing the number of steps the user has to perform. The medication profile provides a useful starting place to perform these actions.

Despite the potential to decrease error, batch processing also introduces an element of increased risk. Medications, diagnoses, allergies, pharmacies, and more are presented in lists, and errors occur as a result of misclicked choices. The same potential for error is introduced with batched processing. An order might be discontinued, refilled, or printed inappropriately.

Direct Editing

Many e-prescribing applications consider a prescription unalterable after it is authorized, yet there is often a need to add or edit certain aspects of the prescription after the fact.

 This nontransmitting information isn't required for dispensing the medication but does add value when it's included. For example, adding an annotation to the prescription describing the patient's experience with the medication (good or bad) could be done after prescribing. Medications may initially be ordered without any relationship to a diagnosis. How should the record be corrected after prescribing? Keeping a portion of the medical order available for appropriate changes after prescribing facilitates organization of the patient record.

 Designer Details

Application designers should allow the user to select a patient's active medication, then choose from a drop-down list populated by the patient's active problems to create a relationship between the medication and the problem. Even better, allowing the association with multiple problems as some medications will affect two or three disease states.

Print Options

The Joint Commission has made medication reconciliation familiar to clinicians in hospital systems. Patient medications must be reconciled at the time the patient enters the hospital and on discharge. The premium placed on the patient's active medication list has never been higher, and the primary care provider's medication profile for that patient holds key information. The ability to print a patient medication list serves dual purposes, both related to patient safety:

 Medication Reconciliation: A hard copy medication list is needed for clinicians without access to an integrated healthcare application. Whether it's faxed from the office, mailed, or carried over by hand, the ability to print and manipulate the patient's active medication list in an efficient fashion is critical to many healthcare processes.

Patient Copy: A hard copy medication list is needed for the patient to carry with him or her—it's a good safety practice. A patient carrying a list of current medications on his or her person is in a much better position in the event of an emergency than a patient without.

 Designer Details

The ability to print an active patient medication list is essential. In order to reduce the potential for error, great care and thought should be put into the design of the reports. Designers should consider creating two reports: one

(continues)

Designer Details *(continued)*

for clinicians and one for patients. Both reports should be formatted such that active medications and directions for administration are clearly presented and unambiguous. In addition, the patient medication list should be printed in a manner that allows for easy storage and transportation in a wallet or purse. Designers should consider formatting the report to print lengthwise on a half sheet of paper (both sides). The blank half can be discarded while the printed half folds accordion-style into approximately the size of a business card. Other formats can be used with a full sheet but require more intricate folding patterns to achieve the necessary size for convenient transportation.

Manipulating the Data

Screening medications for formulary and clinical alerts during prescribing is a proactive process, narrow in its application. To be truly useful, the same tools should be applied retrospectively. At the very least, an option to manually run these important clinical decision support functions should be present.

- *Formulary Alerts:* What if the patient's insurance changes? Will the application generate alerts of medications that have changed formulary status?

  Some applications provide a passive alert in the form of a change in the formulary status tags of the existing medications. An active process would inform the user that a patient's prescription has changed formulary status instead of passively waiting for someone to notice the difference. Proactively addressing formulary changes is good from a prescriber–patient relationship perspective—patients generally like to save money.

  Pushing the boundaries of formulary alerts allows the possibility of displaying projections of the patient's drug expenses due to monthly co-pays, three-month co-pays, and annual expenses. In addition, incorporating Medicare D-specific logic would assist providers in evaluating the impact of drug choice for patients with Medicare D where the best choice is not always obvious. For example, there are some generic medications that enjoy a preferred formulary status though the ingredient cost may be higher than a nonpreferred brand. Because of the way some Medicare D plans are structured, the medication with the lower ingredient cost, though it has a higher co-pay, may be a better economic choice for the patient over the course of the year.

- *Medication History and Drug Interactions:* If a medication that causes a drug interaction is populated into the medication history from an infrastructure provider such as RxHub or SureScripts, will an interaction alert be generated outside of the prescribing process? At least having the option to manually run clinical alerts should be present.

Running the clinical alerts on prescriptions is especially important in the integrated healthcare environment. When more than one prescriber is writing orders on a patient, getting a snapshot of the interaction burden is important for making therapeutic decisions. For example, warfarin may be titrated by a specialist to account for simvastatin's effect. Recognizing that interaction before discontinuing simvastatin in favor of pravastatin could mean the difference between subtherapeutic anticoagulation and appropriately managing a retitration of warfarin.

Medication Renewals

Accessibility

The majority of prescriptions processed in the primary care office are medication renewals, while specialists tend to generate more new prescriptions, according to the specialty. The workflow to process these renewal requests relies heavily on assistants, from the secretary to the medical assistant to the nurse. Assistants own the renewal process in many physician offices as much as prescribers own the process of creating new prescriptions. The eRx NOW application recognizes this division of labor in the placement of the renewal function within the assistant role.

Accessibility Enhancements

Regardless of application, both prescribers and assistants need access to the renewal function as workflows vary from practice to practice. The function should be prominent and intuitive across the application interface.

Some e-prescribing applications have a patient interface through the internet or telephone.[74] The request for renewal is delivered directly to the prescriber for approval.

Designer Details

Making the renewal function assignable as part of a role designation adds flexibility to the process of configuring users.

Renewal Workflow

Once the assistant determines that a medication needs to be renewed, a number of tasks ensue. The ability of the e-prescribing application to efficiently carry the assistant through those tasks (shown in **Table 3.2**) affects the safety of the system. An application that condenses these steps into the fewest number of intuitive and necessary actions will, through the principle of reducing complexity, reduce the potential for error in the system. For example, can searching for a patient and selecting the patient be combined into a single action when sufficient detail is given to make a unique match? Can the act of renewing the order and selection of a disposition (printer, pharmacy, prescriber) be merged? Can multiple orders be renewed at the same time?

The eRx NOW application allows sorting by the date the prescription is written and by medication name; both active and inactive medications are represented. The ability to renew based on an inactive medication saves time when handling periodic therapies such as antibiotics.

Renewal Workflow Enhancements

The same principles of presentation that applied to the medication history also apply to the renewal process. Orders should be displayed in a large font and appropriately spaced to prevent confusion with other orders. Relevant details such as dose, patient instructions, quantity dispensed, refills, days supplied, and pharmacy used should be visible. The enhancements regarding filters for viewing discussed under the medication history apply here as well.

Delightful Displays

Flexible display options are needed for the medication renewal process. Consider the ability to filter by diagnosis and work directly with a patient's diabetic regimen or filtering by a particular pharmacy when renewing maintenance medications.

TABLE 3.2 Assistant Tasks

1. Search for patient record.	5. Verify the order's integrity.
2. Select patient.	6. Renew the order.
3. Access medication history.	7. Select a disposition.
4. Search for the medication order.	

Process

Just as integrated healthcare applications pull together information from various data sources, the e-prescribing application uses its own functions, data, and configuration to define the user's experience. The way these components interact within the application need to be carefully considered. See Chapters 10 and 11 for more information on this subject.

For example, the clinical alerts settings may directly affect the workflows of the assistant and prescriber. Does an alert for an assistant automatically direct the prescription to the prescriber for authorization? What happens if the clinical alerts settings are turned off? Does this allow for unintentional prescribing by an unauthorized person? Regardless of the particular e-prescribing application used, this interconnectedness of functions serves as a reminder to thoroughly test and understand the application's capabilities.

Process Enhancements

The ability to select multiple medications for renewal is an important, nearly essential feature. The iterative process of renewing prescriptions through an entire profile is slashed to a single task of selecting the relevant orders and executing the renewal command.

Another potentially useful feature is an alert flag for medications coming due for renewal. Some offices are better than others at follow-up, but nearly every office has patients who should have been seen and for whatever reason weren't. A reminder of prescriptions coming due for renewal may also serve as a reminder to schedule an appointment for the patient. If we took the reminder a step further, the e-prescribing application might provide the option to generate a patient reminder letter for mailing or e-mail.

Be Wary of Contrary Conventions

Having consistency in the conventions used by the application is underappreciated but so critical to the user's ability to operate the application safely.[64] Does the button labeled "Go" on one screen perform the same action as the button labeled "Done" on another screen? Adherence to common conventions is important. The Tab key advances the cursor to the next logical field; the Return (or Enter) key activates the expected action; clicking an item with the mouse selects it instead of performing an action.

When these conventions are broken or changed, the user becomes confused. It is very disconcerting to press the Tab key and, instead of advancing the cursor to the next field, the prescription is accepted. Different or nonstandard conventions are a significant source of potential error.

Color Confusion

Ferreting out the source of error can be especially challenging when dealing with integrated systems. Consider this illustrative case:

A hospital decided to provide color-coded wristbands for all its patients—red bands for allergies, blue bands to indicate do-not-resuscitate status, and yellow bands to indicate isolation precautions. Every patient status had a corresponding color. All hospital staff underwent in-service training, and the system appeared to be working. Then a patient arrived from another hospital wearing a blue band—but that hospital used blue for its isolation precautions. Another patient came through the emergency room wearing a yellow wristband in support of his brother in Iraq. The hospital's color-coding program had to be abandoned. In isolation and within the self-contained environment, it functioned well. When the internal conventions were placed into the context of the rest of health care and the community, the potential for error blossomed.

The e-prescribing application should be internally and externally consistent. Hyperlinks need to go someplace (some applications have text formatted to look like a hyperlink, but it does absolutely nothing). Buttons should be labeled consistently according to their functions. Contextual hint menus should be employed liberally to orient the user to the intended function of the application's elements.

Bear in mind that every e-prescribing application functions in a specific environment, and no application will perfectly meet the needs of every environment into which it is inserted. The robustness and flexibility of the application will lend themselves to user modification and adaptation in order to meet the unmet needs. For example, one work-around exported an application's prescription summary into an Excel database to create a rolling estimate of prescriptions coming due. Applications can and will have their functions extended by the needs of the work environment. When portions of an application become repurposed, the feature acquires a meaning unique to that work environment and the potential for error rises.

An example of the potential for this repurposing exists in eRx NOW (see Figure 3.3), although other applications also have this potential. When viewing a patient's medication history, a selected order can have a number of actions performed on it. It can be printed, marked as entered in error, discontinued, or marked as completed.

Since these actions alter the status of the prescription, it's important to understand the three ways the medication history is displayed:

1. *Active:* The view displays only prescriptions the patient should be taking as prescribed.
2. *Inactive:* The view displays only past prescriptions the patient should not be taking currently.
3. *All:* The display shows all prescriptions regardless of status.

Now that we have discussed the way the historical view changes depending on the status of the prescription, we can examine what these functions really do.

- *Print:* Selecting this action sends the selected prescription to the printer.

- *EIE:* Selecting this action attaches the entered-in-error status to the prescription and removes it from the active and inactive views.

- *Discontinued:* Selecting this action marks a prescription as inactive with the description of "D/C."

- *Complete:* Selecting this action marks a prescription as inactive with the description of "Complete."

The actions of Print and EIE are self-explanatory, while the actions of Discontinue and Complete are not. Both Discontinue and Complete perform the same action—marking the prescription as inactive—while differing only in their description.

The Complete action is used for short courses of medications such as antibiotics that become completed at the end of their natural course. In contrast, the Discontinue action is used for medications whose natural course was interrupted, such as a dose change.

On further examination, choosing the correct term can be difficult. When a prescriber increases a dose, does that mean the previous order is completed or discontinued? On one hand, the previous dose served its function well until the disease progressed to the point where a higher dose was indicated—the course of therapy at a lower dose is complete. On the other hand, the patient requires an increased dose of the same drug—should the previous dose be discontinued? Medications can be stopped or altered for a variety of reasons including patient preference, adverse effects, formulary rules, fluctuations in disease state, government warnings, manufacturer's availability, and more.

 In reality, the distinction between complete and discontinued carries little clinical significance, depending almost entirely on the subjective interpretation of the user's understanding of those terms and how they relate to the situation at hand. It is a laudable attempt to provide information about the reason for discontinuation, but it can increase the potential for error if the labels are repurposed.

Another danger is the extension and repurposing of those definitions. Assume a primary care office does create and adhere to definitions for complete and discontinue. The term *complete* is used to designate the completion of a therapy for an active patient problem, while *discontinue* is used for failed therapies. Within the medical office, this functions as a useful communication tool, but what of the integrated application? Do these terms communicate their full meaning to other healthcare professionals outside the medical office? What if the integrated application other prescribers use has only one inactive state, or other prescribers choose to use only one action to inactivate medications, or other prescribers have different definitions entirely? The primary care office might erroneously conclude that some therapies, managed by other providers, are failed. Without a common understanding of the conventions used, the use of vague descriptors communicates little of clinical significance at best, and promotes misinformation at worst.

Every application has its features that lend themselves to repurposing. If business rules are needed, as is often the case, consideration should be given to the effect those business rules have in an integrated environment.

Conclusion

In general, users from assistant to prescriber will encounter the features and functions just discussed. Understanding the capabilities and limitations of these common areas of the e-prescribing application assists in the safe and efficient use of the application.

Chapter 4

E-Rx Anatomy– Prescriber Functions

While this chapter appears to focus on prescribers, it is pertinent to anyone creating a prescription. This includes assistants such as nurses or paraprofessionals who create a prescription on behalf of an authorized prescriber. For the sake of simplicity, this chapter broadens the definition of prescriber to include anyone involved in writing prescriptions even if not specifically authorized to do so independently.

The Write Environment

Where the previous chapter dealt with general aspects of an e-prescribing application and features encountered by assistants, the focus of this chapter is on the features and functions that enable the prescriber to generate prescriptions. The same caveats regarding eRx NOW screen shots described in Chapter 3 also apply here and in Chapter 5.

The following three elements come together in an e-prescribing application to allow prescription generation: environment, information, and disposition.

1. *Environment*: The application must provide a comfortable environment for the prescriber to write in that includes patient demographics, the medication history, and prescribing functions.

2. *Information*: The e-prescribing application needs access to various databases to provide information when it's needed: when selecting medications, when providing formulary information, and when displaying previously entered orders. This information also supports features that provide patient education, drug information, and clinical alert documentation.

3. *Disposition*: Something has to be done with the prescription once it's created, such as sending it to the pharmacy, printer, assistant, or storing it in the record.

The eRx NOW application meets these requirements through a variety of prescribing options: prescribing by diagnosis, by favorites (remembered orders), by medication, and free text. This flexible approach allows prescribers the freedom to write prescriptions in a way that suits their patients and practice best. Different pathways to the prescription have corresponding advantages and disadvantages with respect to efficiency and patient safety.

Paper versus Electronic

The process of drug selection is an area where the potential for error is greatest. If nothing else were improved but this, patient safety would still be significantly enhanced. Writing a prescription is very different from electronically creating a prescription. Current e-prescribing applications try to mimic the process that occurs when writing a prescription rather than recognizing the processes that occur when interacting with an electronic medium.

When writing a prescription on paper, the prescriber rarely writes for a different drug by accident. The drug is firmly fixed in his mind and the pen creates the written symbols that communicate what that drug is. Using a pen and paper is a creative process. The first task is to reproduce the name of the drug in a physical form.

When writing an e-prescription, the prescriber fixes the drug in his mind and typically chooses the drug from a list of choices displayed. This is not a creative process; this is an analytical process. The ability of the prescriber to choose the correct drug is limited by his ability to differentiate between a list of choices that may vary only by dose and formulation. An active process occurs as the prescriber compares the image in his head with those listed on the screen; this process doesn't happen on paper. E-prescribing is most successful when it stops trying to mimic paper processes and uses the tools natural to the electronic medium to help the prescriber find the right drug the first time. When that happens, patient safety increases.

> **Designer Details**
>
> The same look-up process for finding drugs should be applied to looking up allergies. It makes the process consistent, causes less confusion, and decreases training needs.

The following strategies may be implemented by e-prescribing vendors to enhance the drug search. Our goal: first drug = right drug.

Prescribing by Diagnosis

Some e-prescribing applications allow the prescriber to identify the indication for the prescription during the prescribing process.[71] Others allow entry of problems or diagnosis independent of the prescribing process. Incorporating the indication or problem into the prescribing process can reduce the number of drugs displayed.

Conceptually, prescribing by first choosing a diagnosis has great appeal. The eRx NOW application has this feature developed to a fuller extent than many other e-prescribing applications. Because the potential benefit—patient safety—is great, it's worth spending some time to explore this feature and workflow further. By the time this book is in print, the implementation of this feature will have changed, but the principles that underlie its strengths and weaknesses will remain.

The workflow in brief follows: The prescriber selects a diagnosis from a list of diagnoses previously used to prescribe medications. If the diagnosis isn't in the list of remembered diagnoses, it must be searched for and selected. Once selected, the application displays medication orders previously written by that prescriber for that diagnosis **(Figure 4.1A)**. If the desired medication order isn't present, the application allows medication entry as usual. The order thus generated is remembered and attached to that diagnosis. The next time the prescriber chooses that diagnosis, the prescription will appear in the list along with other prescriptions written for that diagnosis **(Figure 4.1B)**.

There are benefits to using a diagnosis to drive prescribing:

- The process acts as a soft-forcing function during prescribing. The application displays previous medication orders associated with the diagnosis and excludes irrelevant orders.

- The relationship between medication and diagnosis is created while updating the active medication and problem lists. Both the medication

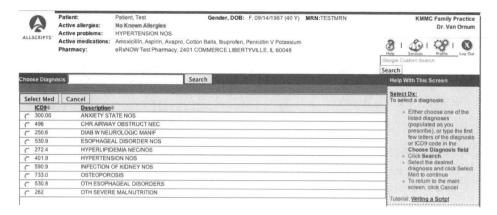

FIGURE 4.1A Choose Diagnosis
Source: Copyright 2007 Allscripts.

history and medication renewal views derive enhanced value from that relationship.

At first glance, the ability to write by diagnosis is efficient with safety benefits both for the prescriber writing the prescription and for other healthcare workers viewing the patient's profile in the future. On second glance, workflow challenges appear. The search process for a diagnosis is cumbersome and unintuitive, drawing from the description tables of ICD-9 codes, which don't reflect vernacular clinical designations. The goal of rapidly finding the desired diagnosis has yet to be reached. Once a diagnosis is chosen, the application displays orders attached to the diagnosis. A single drug can be prescribed in a variety of ways with each unique order becoming stored, making selection of the desired order challenging. For example, different doses are used for warfarin.

FIGURE 4.1B Choose Medication
Source: Copyright 2007 Allscripts.

Example

The prescriber selects the diagnosis of hypertension for a patient, and prescriptions for lisinopril and amlodipine appear. The prescriber writes for felodipine. The next patient also has hypertension that needs a prescription. This time, prescriptions for lisinopril, amlodipine, and felodipine appear when hypertension is selected.

Scrolling through a list of similar orders that vary in only minor details increases the potential for error and is time consuming. Searching for the medication order directly, as is done during the direct medication search, may be safer, but it bypasses the potential benefits of prescribing by diagnosis.

Conceptually, prescribing by diagnosis shows promise for safety and efficiency. Practically, the implementation needs to be refined to the point at which the safest way to enter an order is also the easiest way.

Prescribing by Diagnosis Enhancements

Prescribing by diagnosis may be enhanced by minimizing the use of the search function. When the information is already present, the most efficient solution is to ensure it's displayed when needed. Using the patient's active medication list in an active fashion saves steps. For example, the application could allow the user to summon the order select screen when clicking a diagnosis in the patient header area. When prescribing by diagnosis is chosen, the user could give the patient's existing diagnoses preferential status in the sort list of previously used diagnoses. Most new prescriptions are written for a patient's existing diagnosis as opposed to an entirely new diagnosis. Placing the most frequently used orders at the top of the list rounds out this proposed enhancement.

Increasing the depth of medication–diagnosis relationships is another way to drive utility in this process. When a medication is appropriate for more than one diagnosis, the ability to assign primary and secondary diagnoses treated adds further value to the application. Perhaps the diltiazem for a given patient is for blood pressure *and* heart rate control. Perhaps the paroxetine is for depression *and* anxiety. Making these relationships transparent to other healthcare providers is important for good patient care.

Applications should improve the recognition and retrieval of diagnoses. Allowing the user to create a custom description that is linked to the diagnosis is a useful feature of some applications. The original ICD-9 code is preserved for integrated EHR applications while allowing the clinician to use more familiar abbreviations such as CHF, CAD, and HTN. If these custom descriptions can be shared among practitioners through higher-level integrated applications, a common bridging standard that helps to minimize confusion and error may emerge.

➕ **Applications should increase the breadth of provider–diagnosis relationships.** It is not uncommon to have the cardiologist and endocrinologist contribute to the patient's active medication list. Identifying other prescribers responsible for managing particular diagnoses and problems is another need most acutely seen in the realm of the integrated EHR application. When healthcare workers view the electronic record, how will they know to whom to address their concerns? Identifying the specialist or practitioner involved is a step toward addressing that issue.

Prescription Writing by Favorites

The most convenient method of prescribing in most applications is to choose the medication directly. Searching by medication name in eRx NOW triggers separate processes that follow each other; a list is displayed to allow the selection of a favorite order **(Figure 4.2)**. If the term doesn't find a match, the search is expanded to search for the drug itself. The use of favorites enhances the prescription-writing process in the following two ways: less reentry and less cluttered selection.

⚠ *Less Reentry:* **The work of searching for the medication, the proper dose, patient instructions, quantity dispensed, and refills is already done, saved as a template for future prescriptions.** If a user searches for an order and the favorite is a perfect match, the user can move directly to choosing where to send the new prescription. (Users should check their e-prescribing application for the elements retained in a favorite order. Different vendors create favorites according to their own logic.)

⚠ *Less Cluttered Selection:* **Favorites that match a search criteria are less numerous than a direct medication search.** A search for ciprofloxacin may bring up all the intravenous, oral, ear, and eye formulations along with all possible strengths. The favorites list may have a few orders for oral tablets and the eye drops, reflecting usual prescribing habits. The chance of inadvertently choosing an incorrect formulation is less when using favorites.

⚠ **Favorites minimize, but do not eliminate, the same errors as choosing a drug from a list of drugs.** Unfortunately, their efficiency backfires when errors in the original favorite become propagated across many patients until the error is corrected. Also, the risk of inadvertently selecting the wrong favorite order is still present. Finally, the list of favorites grows over time.

✖ **Like a bush that needs pruning, periodic maintenance may be needed to keep the proliferating orders under control.**

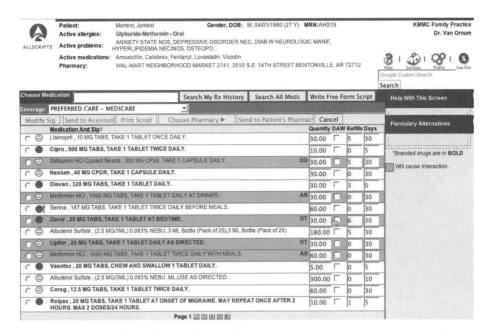

FIGURE 4.2 Medication Selection by Favorites

Source: Copyright 2007 Allscripts.

Common, Frequent, Favorite, Remembered, and Bookmarked Orders

The use of common orders is a great safety benefit for the prescriber, though implementation across applications varies greatly in appearance. Since the eRx NOW application refers to these common orders as *favorites*, and that is the term visible in the screen shots, that is the term used in this book to avoid confusion.

Prescription Writing by Favorites Enhancements

A useful feature in pharmacy and hospital computerized physician order entry (CPOE) applications is the batch order set. In the hospital setting, this feature provides a collection of standard orders based on a given procedure such as a total knee replacement surgery. The concept in primary care is similar—bundle the favorites into logical groupings. Not only does this ensure that appropriate drugs are less likely to be overlooked, but it speeds up the prescribing process.

Beautiful Batches

Orders for opiates to treat chronic pain can be paired with an appropriate bowel regimen. A combination therapy regimen for *Helicobacter pylori* can be prescribed with a grouping of less expensive components.

The favorites list is commonly sorted alphabetically. **Applying a sort order according to frequency of use places the prescriber's most common favorites in a preferred position.** This minimizes selection of the wrong order when the desired order is consistently placed on the screen.

Controlling the organization of the favorites list is important from an administrative level, especially for larger organizations that wish to drive consistency across an integrated application. The ability to import favorites into the e-prescribing application from standard libraries should be evaluated. From where might the orders in these libraries come? Perhaps professional organizations such as the American Heart Association, which already publishes guidelines, would publish a favorites library that contains their recommendations. Insurers often reject orders at the pharmacy as a result of their own **drug utilization review (DUR)**. Perhaps insurers would publish order sets to facilitate cost-effective prescribing.

Organizational Opportunity

Driving drug selection by indication is an opportunity for professional organizations to collaborate on specific therapy suggestions that span multiple disease states. Their suggestions could be incorporated into the e-prescribing application to help the prescriber find the right prescription the first time.

Direct Medication Selection

When a search for a medication fails to produce any favorites, a search for the medication directly ensues. This challenges the e-prescribing application to display the right medication quickly. The robustness of the search logic dictates the success of the application.

Searches that allow for name only tend to overproduce irrelevant results. A good search function will examine different fields (such as name and dose) for matches to narrow the results. Even better are search engines that cross-reference brand and chemical names. The eRx NOW application utilizes a combination-partial search **(Figure 4.3)**.

Search and Display

Once the search is entered, the application needs to display the results. A crowded, jumbled page of results increases the opportunity for error. Search results that are clear and unambiguous are ideal. Readable fonts, relevant columns, and intuitive layouts are hallmarks of a good application and key to minimizing the potential for error that occurs at this step.

The most frequent e-prescribing error is wrong dose.[16,46] Wrong formulation selection is not far behind. For example, chewable tablets are ordered instead of capsules, or tablets are ordered instead of suppositories. The quality of the search results display has direct bearing on the potential for improper formulary selection. To minimize unwanted formulations, use fragments of both drug name and dose (where supported). Different formulations often have different strengths associated with them. Thus, entering *cip 500* in an application that supports a combination-partial search will produce ciprofloxacin 500 mg tablets and avoid the ophthalmic and intravenous formulations.

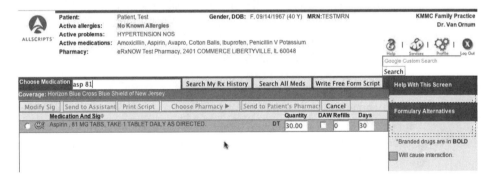

FIGURE 4.3 Partial Search

Source: Copyright 2007 Allscripts.

 Testing Tip

Search for aspirin 325 mg using a variety of methods: asp (to see if it performs a basic partial-letter search), asp 325 (to see if it performs a combination-partial search), asa (to see if it recognizes vernacular abbreviations), and rin 25 (to see if it performs a complex combined partial search). If you are evaluating e-prescribing applications, look for one that supports search logic according to your style.

Search and Display Enhancements

✚ **Incorporating the clinical alerts into drug selection is another strategy with great potential. Already, the formulary status displays next to medications indicating which the payer prefers.** The same kind of dynamic presentation is needed with respect to allergies, therapeutic class, route, contraindication, and indication. The eRx NOW application has this logic implemented with allergies, therapeutic duplications, and drug interactions (see Figure 4.2).

Allergies: In the medication selection list, flagging medications that may cause an allergic reaction identifies selections that will trigger an active alert, thus allowing the prescriber to make an alternate choice. This drives efficiency into the drug selection process.

Therapeutic Class: What if the application user can't remember the name of the specific drug but does know others in the same class? Context-specific JITI, where selection of the drug triggers a display of therapeutic alternatives in another portion of the screen, is one solution. This already happens in a limited fashion when selection of a nonformulary drug prompts a display of the insurance plan's suggested alternatives. Unfortunately, this feature is currently absent for patients whose insurance is unknown, for those who pay cash, or for those who have a plan that doesn't provide this information.

Route: Grouping medications together by route with preference given to the most common routes may minimize wrong-formulation selections. Many applications sort their display based on the drug name and dose, which leaves oral, IV, topical, otic, and compounding preparations to jostle each other on the screen. The difference between an error and the correct medication is about 5 mm on the computer screen.

Indication: Similar to therapeutic class, this display provides a list of medications and formulations indicated for the diagnosis or problem being treated, assuming a problem or diagnosis was specified prior to searching for the drug.

Contraindication: Sometimes concomitant diseases and other medications preclude the use of a particular drug. Identifying drugs meeting contraindication criteria warns the prescriber *before* the drug is selected, not after, as is commonly done. This filter combines logic from the most severe drug interaction checks and incorporates severe drug–disease interactions to drive its alerts.

Patient's Out-of-Pocket Expense: Although it is not a clinical alert, displaying the patient's total monthly cost in the patient header provides a useful basis of comparison. The patient's cost has a significant effect on his or her adherence. Incorporating patient cost into the drug selection process quantifies the incremental addition of expense the drug adds to the overall financial burden.

Not all of these filters should be applied at the same time; rather the technology should have the capability to support these filters. Prescribers will find certain presentations more suited to their practice than others. Regardless of implementation, the principle is the same: preventing the wrong drug or wrong formulary selection in a prospective fashion is preferable to relying on an alert after the drug has already been selected.

Redesigning the Process

Prescriptions are traditionally written by hand with the drug name as the first element written; therefore, e-prescribing applications begin with the prescriber choosing the drug. But is this really the best way?[72]

Since the majority of prescriptions managed in primary care are oral medications, an option to prefilter search results based on oral medications is helpful. Using a route filter minimizes the chance of prescribing ear drops, eye drops, or an intravenous formulation for oral use. Having the prescriber select a route and indication, then using those choices to filter the medication search results is a powerful tool for presenting the right medication the first time and could reduce the number of wrong formulation errors seen.

Right Route

Using the route to drive prescribing is particularly valuable for specialists. The dermatologist could set the default route for topical medications. The ophthalmologist could set the default route for eye medications.

Proactive Filters

Medications have FDA-approved indications. These can be used, in conjunction with the patient's active problem list, to provide dynamic filtering during the prescribing process. For example, starting a prescription for hypertension would present orders previously used by the prescriber for hypertension, followed by medications with FDA-approved indications for hypertension.

Taking this one step further, the application would take into account concomitant disease states such as diabetes, coronary artery disease, or congestive heart failure and present preferred medications that meet the most number of indications, excluding medications the patient is already using. In the example of diabetes, CAD, and CHF, the angiotensin converting enzyme inhibitors would certainly assume priority over agents such as alpha blockers.

Shifting Workflows

An unnoticed and insidious effect of e-prescribing is the delegation to the prescriber of a function previously performed by pharmacists—selection of formulation. With paper prescriptions, the prescriber simply writes the name of the drug and dose. In the e-prescribing application, the formulation is integrated into the drug selection and the options rival those of fast food chains. Would the prescriber like capsules, tablets, or caplets? Would he like the sprinkle form or liquid gel tab? Should he choose extended release, sustained release, controlled delivery, or immediate release?

How does this relate to patient safety? When a prescriber indicates a specific chemical entity and form, the pharmacist has a professional obligation to satisfy the prescriber's intent with a product that meets what is prescribed. **With e-prescriptions, it is often unknown if the choice of formulation is intentional.** If capsules are on the shelf and the prescriber ordered tablets, the pharmacist may call to verify the formulation. If the prescriber gave directions to the patient to take a half dose for the first week, a capsule won't work.

Pharmacists play an important supportive role in the prescription-writing process. E-prescribing needs to preserve the ability of the prescriber to allow the pharmacist flexibility in choosing a formulation when it's appropriate to do so.

Inefficient Infusions

For example, in home infusion a prescription may specify gravity administration of an antibiotic when the homecare standard for that drug is an intravenous bolus administration. If the drug and dose alone are specified, the best formulation to meet the patient's needs can be prepared, taking into account the ability of the patient to learn, infection risks, and administration convenience for the patient.

Custom Medications

What does one do when the medication one wants to prescribe isn't in the application? Searching for a medication can turn up a blank display despite the efforts of the e-prescribing vendor to provide a comprehensive medication database. In this situation, many e-prescribing applications allow the prescriber to enter a drug name as free text. The custom medication order is the do it yourself of prescriptions. **Table 4.1** lists the types of medications orders for which a custom order might be appropriate.

➕ **Nondrug prescriptions warrant further discussion. Custom prescriptions used in this way are examples of extending the functionality of the e-prescribing application.** A nondrug prescription can be a work excuse, an order for a lab test, X-ray, or a prescription for a drug holiday. This increases patient safety by providing additional, relevant information in a place accessible in the higher-level integrated application.

An example of a nondrug prescription would be a neurosurgeon who opens an integrated application and sees a prescription for an MRI of the spine ordered by the PCP. During the visit, the patient can be asked whether the test was done or not. Perhaps the MRI was done at a lab that isn't integrated with

TABLE 4.1 Custom Order Prescriptions

Intravenous preparations

Injectable preparations

Supplies

Investigational drugs

Compounded medications

Nondrug prescriptions

Ruining Reports

Before using custom medication orders in creative ways, users should examine what the potential impact is to reports. If e-prescriptions are being tracked, these creative orders will falsely elevate the order statistics.

Also, if these creative custom orders are sent outside the medical office, the prescriber must ensure the receiver understands how to interpret the order *and* the receiving software can appropriately handle the order.

the neurosurgeon's application. Perhaps the MRI isn't the best test for the patient and the neurosurgeon can intervene with a preferred test. Perhaps the test was done the day before, but results haven't been posted yet. Perhaps the patient forgot or decided against having the test done. The neurosurgeon who has this information is in a better position to obtain necessary and relevant exam results or explore the reasons for a patient's nonadherence. Without the knowledge of the PCP's order, the neurosurgeon may have simply ordered another MRI for the patient.

The custom order provides a way to simulate the CANRX standard, even if the e-prescribing application isn't certified for that standard. As a reminder, the CANRX function allows a prescriber to send a message to the pharmacy that a therapy has been discontinued. This is essential when multiple healthcare providers such as home health care, organizations caring for the mentally retarded and developmentally disabled, home infusion, and elder care are involved. Certain therapies and situations also lend themselves to this feature, including:

- Temporarily stopping an interacting drug while completing antibiotic therapy

- Changing prescriptions in the same day

- Specifying whether a drug is in place of, or added to, a therapy

How can the pharmacist provide appropriate counseling that reinforces the prescriber's instructions to the patient without this information?

The ability to enter medications not found in the database is critical to maintaining the prescribing workflow, yet some overly restrictive applications force the prescriber to write the prescription on paper. Sometimes the application isn't restrictive, but it simply fails to anticipate or hold the information needed. The integrated application suffers the most from this forced change, as the handwritten information is hidden from other healthcare providers. This loss of functionality by the e-prescribing application lays the foundation for future errors.

Custom Medication Enhancements

Certain custom orders are useful and common. If vendors constructed a library of common custom orders, the application would be more useful and contribute to standardization. (Caveat: e-prescribing vendors need to agree on a standard to allow sharing of prescription information. Until then, sharing custom orders is generally restricted to applications by the same vendor.) Like the favorites library, this feature also creates a medium for professional organizations to contribute their expertise to practitioners in the form of custom order templates.

For example, the National Heart, Blood, and Lung Institute (NHBLI) includes oxygen as a recommendation to relieve hypoxia for moderate to severe asthma exacerbations.[79] Oxygen is not usually available as a medication in e-prescribing applications. In the applications where oxygen is absent from the medication list, a custom order is required. If standards for custom orders were in place, the NHLBI could make this order available in a form that provides guidance to the physician while preserving the prescriber's ability to adjust the treatment as needed.

In the context of order sets containing batched orders (as previously discussed), this could potentially allow the prescriber to select asthma as a diagnosis and see the following NHLBI-suggested therapies for moderate exacerbation: beta-2 agonists, systemic corticosteroids, oxygen, and pulmonary function tests.

Formulary Alternatives

Many current applications provide some form of formulary support, as long as a patient has an insurance payer identified as part of his or her profile. During prescribing, selection of a nonpreferred drug may trigger a display of alternate medications the payer would like the prescriber to consider. Whether this display appears depends on the information supplied by the insurance company to the formulary infrastructure provider (see also Chapter 2).

Presentation of formulary alternatives varies depending on the e-prescribing application and insurer. Some applications display a simple alphabetical sorting of alternatives. Other applications present the list from lowest cost to highest cost. Mistaking the list of alternatives as therapeutic equivalents may result in a disastrous error. For example, one application lists methadone as an alternative to sustained-release oxycodone—a potentially fatal suggestion in certain circumstances.

Formulary Alternative Enhancements

First and foremost, a list of clinically relevant formulary alternatives is needed, sorted by the least expensive drug that most closely approximates the prescriber's intended therapy and which takes into consideration any alerts as well as the prescribed drug's therapeutic class. For example: if Nexium, a brand-name proton pump inhibitor (PPI) with no generic alternatives, is prescribed, the formulary alternatives would suggest omeprazole first (a generic PPI), followed by preferred-brand PPIs such as Protonix and Prevacid, followed by generic histamine type-2 receptor antagonists such as ranitidine and famotidine.

Listing drug costs can be improved by augmenting the patient's true out-of-pocket expense with drug pricing information. Displaying this information removes the ambiguity regarding the impact of drug cost to the patient. Due to the tiered co-pay structures some insurances use, the patient's cost may stay the same regardless of the drug chosen. In that case, the payer's cost should be represented and identified as such.

The list of formulary alternatives consists of prescription drugs, though many medications have OTC alternatives that could be used and are not represented. Choosing from the list of formulary alternatives may not be the most cost-effective choice when OTC drugs are not represented.

Sometimes there is no cost-effective alternative. The patient needs the medication. Period. Many drug companies have programs available to help patients who need their medication but have financial difficulties. In addition, several web sites provide information on programs to help financially challenged patients get needed medications, as shown in **Table 4.2**. An e-prescribing application that links to the discount programs available for the medication is valuable in this situation. In addition, providing a link to a form of the program's requirements would allow the prescriber to print the information in the office. Similarly, if prior authorization is needed, and until electronic prior authorization is available, a link to the payer's required prior authorization form is the next best thing.

TABLE 4.2 Patient Assistance Programs

Web Site	Category
www.needymeds.com	General assistance
www.pparx.org	General assistance
www.rxassist.org	General assistance
www.medicationfoundation.com	General assistance
www.edhayes.com/indigent	For the indigent
www.qdrug.com/sf/	Government-funded assistance
www.ncsl.org/programs/health/drugaid.htm#Summary	State assistance programs
www.nami.org/Content/ContentGroups/Helpline1/Prescription_Drug_Patient_Assistance_Programs.htm	Mental health medications

> ✖ **The addition of more clinically relevant information needs to be done without increasing the number of steps or systems in order to keep the potential for error from increasing.**

Patient Instructions
(Sig: Latin Abbreviation for *Signa*)

A long tradition of Latin abbreviations has carried over from paper prescriptions into the workflows of e-prescribing. The same errors made when misreading or misunderstanding an abbreviation are likewise carried over. Most e-prescribing applications are compliant with the Joint Commission's recommendation of abbreviations to avoid and make changes such as substituting daily for QD.[80]

> ⚡ **E-prescribing applications use Latin abbreviations to facilitate the creation of patient instructions in terms with which the prescriber is familiar.** The use of vernacular standard abbreviations helps to create consistency for patient instructions that is easier for the e-prescribing application to manipulate than free-text instructions. At the same time, applications should always make the abbreviation transparent with respect to its full-text meaning in order to promote safety. Examples of this include floating hint text that expands the abbreviation or lists the full text next to the abbreviations.

> ✖ **An unavoidable feature of patient instructions is the free-text field.** There is no way to anticipate the permutations available for patient instructions, and the ability to freely type patient instructions is required in e-prescribing applications for clinical reasons. As a result, the potential for misspellings and grammatical errors exists as when writing on a prescription pad. Some applications compound this error by limiting or truncating the length of the patient instructions allowed. As work on a standard for patient instructions progresses, the need to free text information will migrate into supplementary fields such as Notes for the Pharmacist or Prescription Comments.

> ➕ **A structured Sig is a set of patient instructions the prescriber creates by choosing an application-provided abbreviation.** The application expands on the selection to provide a list of suggested patient instructions. For example, BID could become twice daily, twice daily with meals, one tablet in the morning and one before bed, twice daily before meals, two capsules twice daily, and so on. A very basic application simply provides the literal translation of twice daily into the patient instructions while a more robust application provides medication-appropriate instructions. For example, with carvedilol selected, the application presents "twice daily with meals," since this medication should be taken with food.

Like favorites with medication orders, e-prescribing applications such as eRx NOW can remember preferred sets of patient instructions. These preferred sigs begin with standard instructions associated with the medication, such as the carvedilol twice daily with meals example, and build as the user chooses other patient instructions. Thus, if a prescriber chooses carvedilol three times daily, that becomes an option in the preferred Sig field for future orders, potentially increasing the efficiency of prescribing.

Patient Instructions Enhancements

In 2007, the NCPDP SCRIPT standard transmitted patient instructions as a free-text field, though work is being done to create a standard that would transmit machine-readable patient instructions. The difficulty in establishing the standard is due to the separate growth and maturation of pharmacy and prescribing applications. Pharmacists have long used short codes to rapidly enter patient instructions. These legacy pharmacy applications have their own codes and/or allow the users to develop codes. Pharmacy codes tend to include specific instructions related to administration and food, as shown in **Table 4.3**. In legacy applications, these codes are entered by the pharmacy and are learned almost as a second language by the pharmacist.

The use of codes, however, differs from the growth of e-prescribing mnemonics based on the Latin abbreviations in a mouse-driven environment. The abbreviations are displayed for the prescriber to choose—this is very different than the manual entry the pharmacist experiences in legacy applications grown from a DOS-driven environment. Besides the difference in process, the existence of different sets of codes for patient instructions makes construction of a standard difficult. What would appear in the pharmacy application if an e-prescribing application sent 2DAY, intending 2 tablets daily, while the pharmacist computer interpreted the code as every 2 days? The danger to the patient is great enough that patient instructions must be sent as free text until a standard is approved.

TABLE 4.3 Sample Pharmacy Short Codes

Code	Translation
TIDPC	Three times daily after meals
BIDAC	Twice daily before meals
MEALS	Take with each meal
ACHS	Take before each meal and before bedtime
5D	Take five times daily

General Enhancements

Convergence of functions may find the e-prescribing application capable of supporting orders for blood work, radiography, and consultations. Consolidating the ordering process makes sense given the relationship medications share with other components of the prescriber's armamentarium either to justify therapy or to monitor serum drug levels. Some EMR applications support this crossover functionality, and e-prescribing applications are edging toward that capability with their custom prescriptions. With a few modifications, some e-prescribing applications can already perform these additional tasks.

E-Prescription Destinations

Once the prescription is created, it needs to go somewhere, usually to the pharmacy or to the patient. The options the e-prescribing application presents determine what can be done with the prescription: printing, sending to the pharmacy, sending to another user for processing, or saving it to the profile. Some states require that prescriptions be printed on special paper. Controlled substance prescriptions cannot be sent electronically at this time and must be printed.

A pharmacy must first be selected for the prescription before it can be sent. The e-prescribing vendor provides access (directly or indirectly) to a database of pharmacies capable of receiving electronic prescriptions. If the pharmacy can receive an e-prescription as an EDI transaction, it is sent directly to the pharmacy computer. Otherwise the prescription is sent as a fax transmission. Most e-prescribing applications handle this in the background so the process is nearly transparent to the prescriber.

Many applications will store the patient's pharmacy in memory as part of the prescription or the patient's profile, saving the task of selecting the pharmacy on subsequent renewals. Some applications allow cloning of the prescription for two separate pharmacies. For example, a patient can use a local pharmacy for the first fill and a mail-order pharmacy for maintenance fills.

Disposition Enhancements

With respect to controlled substances, some applications have rules that prevent e-prescribing. In those applications, the option to send the prescription to the pharmacy is removed. There are other circumstances that require a printed prescription, such as New York State's Medicaid law for brand-medically necessary medications. Another situation is a patient who insists on receiving paper prescriptions. Regardless of the circumstance, the ability to extend the forcing function already present could prevent prescribers from inadvertently sending these e-prescriptions that require an inked signature. Applying a state-specific profile of rules is beneficial for prescribers near state lines who write prescriptions in more than one state.

Depth and flexibility need to be added to the choice of prescription destinations. Sometimes a pharmacy is not in the list to be selected. How is it added? Sometimes a prescription needs to go places other than a pharmacy, such as to the payer, patient, or nursing agency. How can the information be sent to those entities? A legal copy for these other recipients isn't always needed. Can the application produce nonlegal copies?

The ability to send the prescription to more than one pharmacy at a time is important and should be further developed by vendors. Initial prescriptions are generally written for a 30-day supply with no refills while maintenance prescriptions are written for a 90-day supply with three refills. Many payers have DUR logic that prevents or hampers the ability of prescriptions for the same drug to be filled at the same time. Ideally, the maintenance prescription should be queued for prescriber approval 20 days later. This supports the prescriber's decision to use a short course of therapy to assess the patient's tolerability. Delaying the transmission of the maintenance prescription allows the prescriber to evaluate whether the prescription is still needed before releasing it to the mail-order pharmacy.

Some insurance payers have preferred pharmacies for specialized therapies such as self-injectables, home infusion, oncology, and HIV medications. Incorporating these preferred pharmacies into the formulary and pharmacy information already supplied may help prescribers send the prescription to the right place the first time.

Samples are discussed more fully in Chapter 5, but aspects of their disposition are worth mentioning here. First, whether a prescription is dispensed as samples should be an option that is both independent of, and in addition to, the traditional options. Second, the dispensing of samples should prompt (or automatically perform) the printing of a drug label and patient information since these components are usually supplied by the pharmacy.

Information

The eRx NOW application contains patient information that can be printed out, professional information in the form of clinical alerts, and an embedded Google search option for internet searching that automatically populates with the currently selected medication or order. The option to print patient medication information is integrated into the prescribing process.

JITI is one of the greatest benefits of e-prescribing applications. Most applications provide patient-level drug information, professional-level information, or both. This information is useful as a quick resource for the prescriber, nurse, and medical office assistant.

Information Enhancements

Many clinicians have electronic resources available through relationships with a medical library, educational institution, commercial applications, or saved internet links. E-prescribing applications could import these links or map to a customized information infrastructure, similar to the way a web browser's home page is set, making them accessible to prescribers.

In the same way, patient resources beyond drug information should be accessible through a list of customizable links. For a prescriber who is writing a new prescription for an antihypertensive, expanded links provide access to patient information on the dietary approaches to stop hypertension (DASH). For someone writing a prescription to treat insomnia, expanded links provide access to a sleep diary and information on good sleep hygiene. Developing relationships between the patient-specific information and the drugs themselves is the next step to drive meaningful prompts and to increase JITI during prescribing.

A patient's direct comments could be included in the patient's profile. For higher level integrated applications, the patient's perspective on his or her medications could help other healthcare workers provide care.[81]

Conclusion

Users should be sensitive to the manner in which features that support e-prescribing are implemented. A required e-prescribing feature may be present but implemented so poorly as to be functionally absent or contributing to the potential for error. Other applications may have functions that can be adapted to meet the users' needs in creative ways, such as the custom medication order.

Chapter 5

E-Rx Anatomy– Administrator Functions

 READING PRIORITY

Managing the Details

An administrator sets up and manages users and clinical alert settings and configures other options and features that make the e-prescribing application operate the way it does for a particular user. This chapter is for those individuals taking on the additional responsibility to care for this infrastructure. In addition, we'll cover topics that don't fit well into the previous two chapters.

Administrative Functions

Many administrative functions are application specific, though the features can be generalized into four broad categories as follows and as shown in **Figure 5.1**:

Users: Users need to be added to the application with their roles specified as a prescriber or nonprescriber, any special designations, and relevant demographic information. Once users are added, the administrator can adjust individual settings as needed.

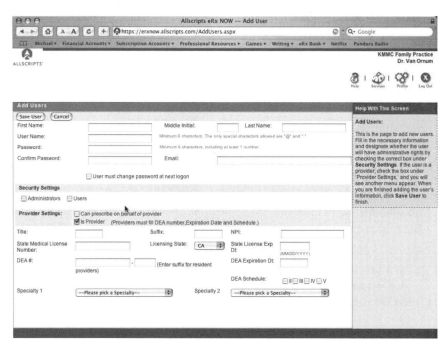

FIGURE 5.1 Administrative Functions
Source: Copyright 2007 Allscripts.

When entering a user in eRx NOW, the prescriber role designation opens another window for prescriber-specific information—minimizing unnecessary information reduces the potential for error (**Figure 5.2**).

Security: These functions include setting and resetting passwords, determining how long the application remains active before logging the user

FIGURE 5.2 Add Users
Source: Copyright 2007 Allscripts.

out, whether a password is required to authorize a prescription, and how many log-in attempts will cause a user to become locked out.

Site: The demographics for the site need to be entered and kept up to date. This information is used by the application to print the office name, address, and phone number on prescriptions. Some situations call for multiple sites to be set up and configured if users prescribe from different locations.

Settings: All the customizable features that affect the user's global experience are set here. In many cases, this includes the clinical alerts. The administrator determines, within the limits of the application, which alerts are triggered during order entry, at what level, and the type of alerts allowed. Other settings may include automatic printing of an office copy of a prescription, the persistence of discontinued orders, and preferences for favorites.

Reports

E-prescribing applications usually have basic reporting abilities for different situations. Three reports should interest nearly every office: the transmission log, recall reports, and report of daily prescriptions written.

Transmission Log: Just as fax machines sometimes have errors when transmitting, e-prescriptions become lost in the electronic web. The transmission log records the final disposition of a prescription. Was it printed? Accepted by the pharmacy? Was there an error? Does the prescription need to be re-sent? Some e-prescribing vendors have an active process to inform users of dropped or corrupted transmissions. Other vendors give users the burden of ensuring the prescription arrived as intended. The potential workflow this represents should be taken into account prior to implementation. See also Chapters 10-12.

Transmission Troubles

When prescriptions aren't transmitted as expected, the user needs tools available to discover the reasons why. Each user should take a moment to become familiar with the transmission report or equivalent process for managing failed transmissions. Can he or she easily trace failed prescriptions back to the patient's profile? Does the report have robust sort and filter options? Does the report provide the level of detail needed to act? If active vendor support is involved, what is the turn-around time?

(Rx) **Pharmacist Perspective**

Automated faxed prescription renewal requests resemble failed prescriptions to prescribers and their staff. Ensure that any automated fax systems are linked to the pharmacy dispensing system such that an automatic fax for a prescription renewal will be cancelled if the prescription has been filled.

In the absence of such communication, the automated fax system may send a renewal request for a prescription the prescriber had sent electronically a few days earlier—the filled prescription may be waiting for the patient to come and pick it up. The prescriber and their staff lose faith in the e-prescribing application and spend unnecessary time and energy resending prescriptions or contacting the pharmacy about the repeat renewal request.

Recall Reports: This report doesn't tell what is recalled, but it does help identify patients who might be taking a recalled drug. For example, when the controversy surrounding rosiglitazone erupted in June of 2007,[82] this report could provide a listing of patients in the practice taking that drug.

Prescriptions Written: From a quality assurance perspective, a report of all the prescriptions written by a prescriber in a given time period is helpful. As discussed in other chapters, the habit of reviewing a daily log of prescriptions written can help to identify errors and allow prescribers to act before harm comes to the patient. In addition, this report can identify someone sending prescriptions without proper authorization.

Other useful reports include a listing of medication changes on a per-patient basis for a given time frame, a listing of agents used for a diagnosis, the percent of generic versus brand drugs prescribed, the frequency of alerts and resulting changes, orders stored as favorites not used in the last 90 days, and the percentage of prescriptions written for specific insurance payers (**Figure 5.3**).

Maintenance

Depending on the application and configuration, the administrator may be called on to perform the maintenance that keeps e-prescribing working in the office. See also Chapters 10-12.

Updates and Upgrades: The administrator may be required to install any needed e-prescribing updates and upgrades in the future.

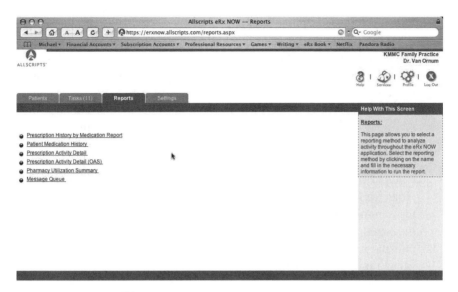

FIGURE 5.3 e-Prescribing Reports
Source: Copyright 2007 Allscripts.

Data Scrubbing: Despite the best intentions, patient data can become corrupt. Duplicate records of patients need to be merged, demographic fields inadvertently become altered, and missing information needs to be filled in.

Pruning Favorites: Absent a mechanism for controlling the proliferation of favorites, the administrator should oversee the routine elimination of extraneous and erroneous favorites.

Technical Troubleshooting: When problems arise, the administrator may be the one making calls to the vendor support desk or troubleshooting the specific issue.

Training: In addition to setting up users in the application, the administrator may train new staff or make a significant contribution to their training.

Disaster Plans: The administrator is often the keeper of the disaster plan when the unexpected makes e-prescribing nonfunctional.

Interface Integrity: The e-prescribing application may exchange data with other healthcare applications such as a practice management system or health information exchange. If there are manual processes involved in maintaining this data sharing, the administrator will likely be involved.

Administrative Enhancements

Site Relationships: Setting up sites and users can be a repetitive, time-consuming task. The usefulness of designating relationships between sites, organizations, practices, and prescribers should not be overlooked.

This level of organization is essential when managing larger groups and when interacting with higher-level integrated applications.

Workflow Relationships: Within the office, designating assistants who work closely with assigned providers aids in tailoring the application to meet the user's needs. Matching an assistant to a prescriber affords the opportunity to selectively filter much of the work of both, resulting in greater efficiency and safety. This kind of relationship is also applicable with special users or guest prescribers such as students, residents, and staff in training.

Automated Tasks: The application can save the administrator time, support office workflows, and ensure that needed maintenance occurs by allowing the administrator to schedule needed reports to run at regular intervals.

Administrator Alerts: Administrator-specific alerts could be used to indicate unusual user activity, failed e-prescribing transmissions, or identifying when a user is locked out of his or her profile.

Tasks and Communication

E-prescribing applications share tasks among users in many ways. The purpose of tasks, assignments, jobs, communications, notes, or whatever designation an application uses remains constant. That purpose is to translate workflows that exist on paper into electronic form. Overall, this increases communication, although poor implementations of this feature strain that assessment. The communication options these tasking functions represent challenge the way information has traditionally passed among prescribers, pharmacies, and office staff.

Prescribers' Perspective

Prescribers' interactions with office staff are highly dependent on context and vary widely from office to office. Prescribers may send prescriptions to assistants that are authorized or approved but need additional attention. Some examples include prescriptions requiring prior authorization, further clarification with the patient or pharmacy, or printed patient instructions.

Assistant Augmentation

The eRx NOW application allows the prescriber the option to send to an assistant during prescribing. The prescriptions enter a queue from which any assistant can open the prescription and follow the established workflow for those tasks. Other applications apply similar functionality according to their design.

Part of the certification of pharmacy applications for e-prescribing ensures that electronic renewals can be sent. In eRx NOW, these pharmacy tasks appear in the same form as assistant requests for renewals or new prescriptions. Other applications may separate the pharmacy-generated renewal requests from assistant-generated requests.

Assistant's Perspective

Assistants play a key role in the prescriptive process by handling most of the prescription renewal requests, fielding patient phone calls regarding medications, and initiating orders for prescribers to authorize.

Example

The eRx NOW application allows assistants to process renewal requests depending on the presence of clinical alerts. If there are no clinical alerts, the prescription is processed. If there are, the prescription is forwarded to the prescriber for review.

If the administrator turns off alerts, all prescriptions may be processed by the assistant on behalf of the prescriber.

Overall, the assistant has fewer options available for communicating directly to the pharmacy through the e-prescribing application; nearly every opportunity passes through the prescriber. Communications from the pharmacy appear in the prescriber's task list and whether the assistant is able to view the request depends on the e-prescribing application.

Task and Communication Enhancements

For the Prescriber

 The prescription has a section for comments designated for the pharmacist. **To accommodate the workflow of many offices, a section to allow directions for an assistant is needed. Table 5.1** lists sample communication topics.

Triggered events during prescribing can be used to enhance communication. For example:

- Overriding an alert might copy the triggered alert and reason for the override into the pharmacist's comment field as part of the prescription.

TABLE 5.1 Assistant Communication Topics

Medication prior authorization
Patient medication information
Patient disease information
Scheduling and confirming follow-up visits
Scheduling lab work and retrieving results
Special administration instructions
First-dose administration

- Prescribing a sample medication sends a prescription to the pharmacy with a notation of "Sample Medication: Do Not Dispense" in the pharmacy communication field. This puts the medication in the pharmacy profile and allows it to be included in pharmacy DUR checks.

- Discontinuing a medication in a patient's profile automatically sends a CANRX to the pharmacy. If the CANRX standard isn't supported yet by the e-prescribing application, a custom prescription communicating the discontinuation may be sent.

For the Assistant

As the front-line recipient of questions and concerns from patients and pharmacies, an assistant needs to have an efficient method of communication in place within the e-prescribing application. For example, a place is needed for the assistant to add a comment indicating the patient is doing well, has a specific complaint, or that a clinical concern exists with the prescription. If the assistant can add the prescription and comments to the prescriber's task list, the information is communicated more efficiently than immediately disrupting the prescriber's work.

Other situations call for direct communication options, such as patient insurance changes or patient vacations. A place to store these assistant-generated nuggets of information needs to be present on the prescription prepared for the prescriber. During the patient visit, the prescriber will be able to adjust new and renewed prescriptions accordingly.

General E-Prescribing Enhancements

While the eRx NOW application has been a useful discussion device, it doesn't contain all features in all e-prescribing applications. This brief section highlights two areas in particular that may benefit users and patients.

Sample Management

Handing out free samples is a labor-intensive, costly service that many offices provide. On the front end, patients are left with an expensive co-payment when their sample runs out. In many cases, the patient either stops taking the medication entirely or returns to the office to ask for more samples. On the back end, office staff may be used to consolidate samples into different dispensing sizes, create labels, and generate instructions. Office staff and prescribers spend more time with pharmaceutical company representatives to obtain the samples, which often translates into less time with patients. The true cost of free samples includes transforming the office into a mini pharmacy and a higher rate of patient nonadherence through increased co-pays. If samples are used, the prescriber should consider writing a prescription for a less expensive alternative; it benefits both the office and the patient.[83-87]

E-prescribing applications are positioned to streamline management of samples through a robust search engine, medication tables, and organization of information. That said, an efficient entry process such as bar codes is needed to log sample lot numbers, package size, and expiration dates.

As discussed in the previous chapter, printing labels and patient medication information when prescribing samples gives the patient information she would normally receive at the pharmacy. Communicating sample distributions to the pharmacist is important. Besides including the sampled drug in interaction checks, it provides the pharmacist a sense of timing. This provides an explanation for gaps in the patient's refill history. The urgency for filling a medication or the window of time for ordering a specialty drug changes if samples have been given. Finally, the pharmacist can provide counseling on the sampled product that supports and enhances the information the prescriber gave the patient.

Incident Reporting and Documentation

There are several national and state reporting mechanisms in place to capture adverse drug events. These mechanisms include MedWatch, Joint Commission sentinel events, and state-mandated reporting. The current process for this reporting activity relies heavily on clinician initiative. For example, a MedWatch report should be completed when a patient reports an unusual side effect that appears to be related to a medication. Unfortunately, the degree of clinician exposure to these programs is variable and the procedure for completing the report is cumbersome. The vast majority of reports actually come from the pharmaceutical industry as opposed to front-line clinicians.

Integrated documentation may make participation in federal programs such as MedWatch easier.[88] Blank report forms for these programs may have an electronic or online presence that could be linked into the e-prescribing application. For example, a patient has taken his medication and calls with a report of a purple rash across his chest. He stopped the medication and the rash went away. He restarted the medication and the rash came back. It sounds like a drug reaction that should be reported—but the paperwork is daunting. The information in the e-prescribing application and HIE could populate a MedWatch report, making it nearly ready for submission. An easier reporting process will help clinicians provide information that improves safety across the nation.

Conclusion

The administrative functions of e-prescribing applications have a front-loaded responsibility; most of the work—setting up users, sites, and determining the initial configuration—is done before or during implementation. When evaluating an e-prescribing application, this preparatory work is important to consider. Someone evaluating an application should take a moment to investigate whether the application contains features that make this initial workload easier. As a close follow-up, that person should evaluate the maintenance work required by the application and who is required to do the work; he or she should determine whether it is spread over all users or concentrated only on the administrator.

PART III

Improving Patient Safety

Chapter 6

E-Prescribing in the Integrated Environment

Co-authored and edited by Marie Smith, PharmD

 READING PRIORITY

Integrated Networks

Regional health information organizations and large healthcare organizations are forming HIEs as an answer to the challenge of improving patient safety by collecting and organizing information from multiple disparate (e.g., physicians, hospitals, labs, pharmacies, payers, and patients) sources on a scale not seen before. This aggregation of clinical data paves the way for advanced clinical decision support in healthcare applications,[89-91] and the potential cost avoidance generated by the HIE's information resource is an important factor in their business plan. Some large, integrated health systems have developed the infrastructure to support clinical data sharing among their affiliated providers; however, the RHIO's infrastructure spans providers regardless of company affiliation. For simplicity, this chapter uses the functional sense of the term *HIE* to include large, integrated health systems, RHIOs, or any other network that collects and disseminates health information on a community scale.

Safety Pays

Medical errors have a significant financial impact on direct costs to the health-care system, employers, and patients as well as indirect costs from lost productivity. In 1997, estimates from the hospital setting placed the cost of an adverse drug event at $2,262[29] and the cost of a preventable adverse drug event at $4,685.[30] For Medicare D recipients, CMS estimates the potential savings in 2009 due to avoided adverse events as a result of prescriber adoption of electronic prescribing to be between $50 million and $149 million.[53]

RHIOs bring together health information from many disparate sectors horizontally and vertically—horizontally in that different hospital systems become linked through the HIE, and vertically in that data from physician offices through large healthcare systems are integrated.

This integration of health records from different sources creates new safety challenges for the e-prescribing application. Creating a medication order that is easy to understand is important not only for the pharmacist, but also for other healthcare professionals who may base clinical decisions on the medication order. In a real sense, the prescription goes both ways (see **Figure 6.1**).

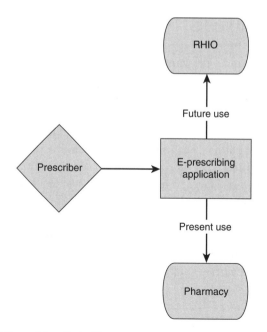

FIGURE 6.1 E-Prescribing Data Flow

This chapter explores the ways RHIOs are organizing data,[92] how that affects e-prescribing, and the potential this interconnectedness has for the patient's safety through promotion of clinical decision support.[93,94]

Pharmacist Perspective

Advanced clinical decision support features are becoming more important to pharmacists for two reasons. First, pharmacies are now sources of information for infrastructure companies such as SureScripts. The second reason is the movement to consolidate healthcare information. Already, clinical pharmacists in many areas of the country have access to these resources through HIE networks. In the future, this information may be delivered directly to the dispensing pharmacists in the form of advanced CDS alerts that complement the current clinical alerts. The availability of relevant health information allows the pharmacist to provide better care.[58]

E-prescribing software with advanced CDS incorporates patient-specific information as opposed to order-specific information utilized by clinical alert functions. Unfortunately, the level of CDS used to write an order is not shared as part of an e-prescription's transaction. The pharmacist must perform all the usual and customary checks to ensure the appropriateness and safety of the prescription. This work flow will not change until e-prescribing vendors standardize CDS processes and disclose the alerts presented, along with the prescriber's response, in a way that is transparent to the pharmacist.

Stand-alone, electronic drug reference tools are sometimes incorrectly considered e-prescribing tools. A more accurate designation would be e-prescribing aids, since they can be useful drug information sources. However, they are not e-prescribing applications and do not offer integrated CDS.

The Challenge

Health data exists in many different places. Hospitals, physician offices, pharmacies, nursing agencies, radiology services, clinics, and laboratory services are examples of data sources, each with its own way of keeping the data organized. The barrier to a community-wide electronic patient record isn't a lack of data but a lack of consistently implemented standards across the health environments.[95] The HIE's task is to unite these sources in a common interface that facilitates information sharing. Patients should not be discounted as active participants,[74,81] though HIPAA concerns must be addressed[26] when patients actively participate.

The following questions, answered by the HIE in general, are also relevant to e-prescribing applications:

- How should the HIE receive and combine the different data types? What are the data sources capable of delivering?

- Can the e-prescribing application deliver data in the right format for the HIE? Are CMS e-prescribing standards being used?

- What information technology expertise is required? How much hardware is needed? How much software? How much ongoing maintenance?

- What kind of interface is needed for the e-prescribing application? Is additional equipment needed?

- What infrastructure will be used to support the data sharing—a federated model in which the HIE acts as a guide for applications to find the data that is needed, or a centralized model in which the HIE combines the data into a central data repository? Or will an entirely different model be used?

- Will e-prescribing data be referenced by the HIE or copied into a central data repository? Does this mean users have to keep a computer on and active for the data to be accessed?

This distillation of standards into a common denominator challenges the way data sources handle and present their data. The HIE needs to work with the data sources on formats that can be manipulated. The search is not for a single interface or even an interface for every data source; it is to get the data into the least number of common standards and conventions as possible.

Creating data streams from large sources of healthcare information to the HIE can be difficult. Most legacy applications in health care were designed to function independent of other applications. For example, a hospital or healthcare system usually has a single application for managing admissions, discharges, and transfers (ADT). The focus of the application is management of ADT events, not communication with other ADT applications. In the same way, most e-prescribing applications are designed to manage prescriptions, not to communicate with other e-prescribing applications or large health systems.

As we saw in Chapter 2, prescription and drug data are affected by multiple standards. In the e-prescribing application, the transmission standard for prescription information is NCPDP SCRIPT. EHRs and EMRs may use CCRs to organize clinical information. A hospital may use the HL-7 standard, though the flexibility of the standard creates significant challenges in reconciling the data.

The decisions of the HIE may place boundaries on what the user can and can't do with integrated data. For example, certain high-level CDS functions require information best manipulated in a CCR form as opposed to a SCRIPT form. The HIE's presentation of the data may be like a portable digital file (pdf) that cannot be edited but only viewed, or a database file in which data relationships exist that can drive expanded functions, or a text file in which the content and appearance may be changed but the data itself lacks organization to drive other functions.

The HIE seeks to collect the patient medication history, problem list, allergies, and demographics from the e-prescribing application. Of the information available, the active patient medication list is the most valuable data that e-prescribing offers the healthcare community from a safety perspective.

If the HIE collects incomplete or inaccurate data, patient safety will decline. As clinicians, we need to understand the data acquisition challenges the HIE faces if we are to provide any assistance, or at least avoid becoming a hindrance. The way we enter information into the e-prescribing system, as well as the quality of information entered, is critical to the integrity of the HIE's information, its usefulness to other clinicians, and by extension, to the safety of the patient.

Active Medication List

Keeping an active medication list sounds simple but can be an amazingly difficult task. The physician records, the pharmacy records, and the patient's records may reveal very different lists. The primary physician may include the OTC medications the patient is taking but not the medications the specialist prescribed.[96] The pharmacy may have prescriptions written by the specialist and primary care physician but not the OTC medications that the patient uses at home. The patient may report variances in the intended therapies as a result of misunderstanding medication instructions or self-treatment with herbal or home remedies. In addition, a patient may be using an outdated OTC product or discontinued prescription that does not appear on any physician or pharmacy list. Therefore, an accurate, active medication list for a patient requires triangulating multiple sources of medication use information from prescribers, pharmacies, and the patient. See also "Patient Medication History" in Chapter 11.

A patient's comprehensive medication list should include the elements outlined in **Table 6.1**.

Here is an example in which an active medication list can be most helpful in the detection of an adverse drug effect and an unnecessary medication:

TABLE 6-1 Active Medication List Elements, Patient Safety Implications, and Sources

Elements	Patient Safety Implications	Data Source Reliability (+) higher reliability (−) lower reliability			
		Pharmacy	**Payer**	**Prescriber**	**Patient***
Prescriptions					
Brand or generic name	Identifies therapeutic duplication, clinical appropriateness, drug interactions, allergies	+	+	+	+/−
Dosage	Allows assessment for underdosing, overdosing, drug interactions, food interactions, contraindications, adverse effects, side effects, pharmacokinetic concerns, potential cost issues	+	+	+	+/−
Route of administration		+	+	+	+
Number of doses per day		+	−	+	+/−
Times of administration		−	−	−	+
Start date and stop date (if discontinued)	Identifies medication as active or inactive, length of therapy	−	−	+/−	+/−
Prescriber's name and contact information	Discuss patient medication problems, adherence issues; identify multiple prescribers	+/−	+/−	+	+/−
Pharmacy's name and contact information	Verify prescription/refills/adherence; identify multiple medications with abuse potential	+	+	−	+
Over-the-Counter Medications					
Elements Same as for Prescriptions Examples: Aspirin, antacids, cough/cold, anti-inflammatory, antidiarrheals, pain medications	Potential drug interactions, therapeutic duplications, side effects, contraindications, allergies	+/−	−	+/−	+

*need to assess patient reliability of information

Herbal Products

Elements Same as for Prescriptions

Examples: St John's wort, echinacea, teas, cultural/home remedies	Potential for drug interactions, therapeutic duplications, side effects, contraindications, allergies	+/−	−	+/−	+

Dietary Supplements

Elements Same as for Prescriptions

Examples: Vitamins, nutritional supplements, garlic, yeast, fish oils	Potential for drug interactions, therapeutic duplications, side effects, contraindications, allergies	+/−	−	+/−	+

DE, an 82-year-old gentleman, saw his urologist for frequent urination and was given samples of long-acting oxybutinin. Two weeks later, DE's wife brought him to see his primary care physician for increased forgetfulness and confusion, along with all his prescriptions. Since the oxybutynin had been sampled in the manufacturer's packaging, the wife neglected to bring it with the pharmacy-supplied medications. Nor did she mention that she had begun giving DE a nighttime dose of diphenhydramine to help him sleep. DE's mini-mental status exam demonstrated cognitive impairment and the physician began donepezil for suspected Alzheimer's disease. DE continued to deteriorate over the next month and a nursing home placement was strongly considered by the family.

If this patient had an active medication list that was accurate, comprehesive, and available to all DE's prescribers, providers, and pharmacies, this situation could have been avoided. Anticholinergic medications such as oxybutynin and diphenhydramine can precipitate significant mental status changes in the elderly. In contrast, donepezil promotes cholinergic activity; this is an excellent example of a drug being prescribed for the side effects of another.

Medication Reconciliation and E-Prescribing

In 2006, the Joint Commission instituted a new national patient safety goal to implement medication reconciliation processes to reduce the number of medication errors that reach the patient.[16] This goal applies to all accredited health organizations throughout the continuum of care—in hospitals, in emergency departments, in home care, and in outpatient clinics.

Medication reconciliation is the process of comparing the medications that the patient has been taking prior to the time of admission or entry to the healthcare setting with the medications that are about to be given or changed as a result of being in the healthcare setting. The process is complex, involves multiple stakeholders, and demonstrates the need to harmonize standards across a variety of healthcare settings.[97] The purpose of the reconciliation is to avoid errors of transcription, omission, or duplication of therapy and to detect potential drug interactions upon admission, transfer, or discharge.

E-prescribing and the development of an active medication list that can be available to all healthcare providers and settings can greatly assist in meeting the safety goal of medication reconciliation. E-prescribing will capture prescription medications ordered from multiple prescribers (primary care and specialist physicians). Pharmacy data will be required to enter the active prescriptions that were filled and picked up by or for the patient. In addition, pharmacy data is the most reliable source of information to assess patient adherence (compliance and persistence).

The patient/caregiver or healthcare professional needs to provide updated medication information of all medications at home (including OTC medications, herbal products, and dietary supplements) so that an accurate, comprehensive, and active medication list can be created.

It is equally important for the patient or a family member/caregiver to always have access to an updated, active medication list. Healthcare professionals should review the patient's current list; record any new, changed, or discontinued medications; and provide an updated, written copy to the patient/caregiver. At home, it is recommended that a patient keep this list for emergency first responders to verify current medications. Patients should carry the most updated list to all healthcare visits (physician, dentist, eye doctor, pharmacy, lab, hospital, emergency department, clinics).

Active Problem and Allergy List

Problem lists or active diagnoses—the terms are sometimes used interchangeably—exist within EMRs and billing applications in addition to some e-prescribing applications. In general, physicians treat active problems and bill for diagnoses. Some institutions will apply algorithms to medical claims to identify probable diagnoses, creating a speculative problem list.

When patient diagnoses are an option in the e-prescribing application, their presence is usually to support prescribing functions and may not represent the breadth of the patient's conditions; not every diagnosis requires a prescription. From the HIE perspective, data from e-prescribing regarding problems and diagnoses confirms and augments information from other systems but rarely suffices as a sole information source.

Allergies may have the richest detail in the e-prescribing application. Not only is the specific allergy present, but the reaction and severity may also be known. See also Chapter 3.

If an e-prescribing application or EMR is supplying data to an HIE or other healthcare information exchange, accurate and complete problem and allergy lists are needed. To improve the quality of the allergy and problem list in an e-prescribing application, one should consider answering these questions:

- If the e-prescribing application has a place for allergies and problems, are they being used?

- If the workflow to use allergies or diagnoses is cumbersome, has someone contacted the vendor about it?

- Are there sources, such as the EMR (if present), that can drive allergies and problems in the e-prescribing application?

- Can allergies and problems in the e-prescribing application populate problem lists in the EMR (if present)?

- Can one use diagnoses to drive efficiency during prescribing?

- Can the billing system be used to populate diagnoses into the e-prescribing application or vice versa?

Patient Safety Depends on Standards

Problem lists and allergies are especially useful to clinicians caring for unfamiliar patients.

❶ **If the HIE chooses a standard that cannot support the level of detail available, patient safety may suffer.** For example, a medication list may be supplied, but without indications. Allergies may be given, but without reactions. The search for the common information standard may eliminate the particular features that differentiate the diverse healthcare information sources and result in a loss of content.

HIE Safety Benefits

The HIE network isn't only a beneficiary of e-prescribing data; it also offers the benefits of networked healthcare systems to the users of an e-prescribing application. These benefits may consist of broad features such as lab results, test results, consultation notes, visit histories, progress notes, and enhanced communication options in various combinations, depending on the capabilities of the HIE network.

Through the HIE, relevant and important information is brought one step closer to aid the prescriptive process. Laboratory results are one example. Some medications are directly monitored through blood sampling. Other medications have dosing that depends on assessments of body functions through blood sampling.

Having these laboratory results accessible at the point of prescribing increases the likelihood they will be referenced, which increases the safety of the process. As Chapter 7 will explore, taking laboratory results directly into the e-prescribing application leads to advanced clinical decision support.

HIE Benefits in Action

Legacy healthcare applications that were never designed to work with each other may find a common ground in the HIE and find their functionality extended or enhanced. For example, an e-prescribing application may send a prescription to the pharmacy and post it on the HIE. This allows a nursing agency involved in the care of the patient to access the prescription. That's one prescription, but two orders; no separate faxing or phone calls are needed. Other benefits include:

- *HIE-Based Messaging:* This messaging allows HIPAA-compliant sharing of patient information among healthcare providers.

- *Facilitated EMR Adoption:* Practices unable to convert to electronic medical records may find interim solutions in the HIE.

- *Increased Patient Safety:* Beyond the benefits to prescribing, the HIE's patient data resource aids the emergency room, specialist, pharmacist, nursing agency, and more. Healthcare providers caring for the patient are able to make better decisions with easy access to relevant information.

Conclusion

The emergence of HIE networks and concomitant demand for integration technology place new requirements on healthcare application vendors. Medical applications should now consider the needs of two customers—the medical office and the HIE network. The ability of the new breed of applications to share data may have direct effects on patient safety and provide a greater incentive for offices to adopt good documentation habits that lead to accurate and complete information.

Chapter 7

Clinical Decision Support

 READING PRIORITY

This chapter has a threefold purpose: to raise awareness of patient safety issues, to identify desirable safety features of e-prescribing applications, and to provide the clinician with a stable of focused questions to ask the application vendor. The questions and testing tips are meant to help users explore the capabilities of their e-prescribing application or as an assessment tool that complements Chapter 8. Users of the application have the power to proactively identify safety features most relevant to their practice. Having an awareness of the potential benefit within the technology allows us to advocate for these features in a manner that guides software developers to bring this potential to reality.

Integrated healthcare applications and their associated data are the foundations on which effective CDS is built. Jonathan Teich outlined a number of features and elements an e-prescribing application should have to deliver effective clinical decision support,[57] and many of these features already exist in various forms within current e-prescribing applications. As with standards, the implementation of these features determines whether it increases safety or the potential for error. This discussion builds on the work of Kuperman and colleagues[75] and Wang[71] to focus on current CDS features, emerging features, and future areas of opportunity related to patient safety.

CDS is present in all areas of the e-prescribing application, though its voice is loudest through its alerts that warn and inform. Unfortunately, it is a voice that fades easily into the background.[98] Alert fatigue causes many clinicians to turn off or ignore the alerts, and it occurs when the number of alerts is great or when the information is not clinically significant. When alert fatigue sets in, the potential for error and patient harm increases. Every effort should be made to reduce alert fatigue or, at the very least, provide the tools to do so.[64-67,73,99,100]

What constitutes a reasonable use of alerts? At least for drug reactions, studies indicate alerts interrupting the workflow should be reserved for true allergies and severe intolerances or hypersensitivities.[77,78]

Current Features

Most e-prescribing applications have the majority of basic CDS functions Teich outlined, though drug utilization review (DUR) functions are worth a few words. Depending on the sophistication of the application, checks on the prescribed order are performed. These include allergy and dose checking, food/drug interactions, drug/drug interactions, and drug/disease interactions.

In 2007, e-prescribing applications had a rudimentary ability to perform these clinical alert checks.[101] Drug interactions are one example. A prescribed drug is compared to a database of known interactions, and the resulting information is displayed to the prescriber.

 There is no adjustment for other information in the patient's profile as the sidebar examples from actual alerts illustrate.

Sample Drug Interaction Alerts

Alert No. 1
Interaction: Furosemide and lisinopril
Severity: Moderate

Effect: Pharmacologic effects of loop diuretics may be altered by ACE inhibitors. Captopril may decrease and ramipril may increase the diuretic and natriuretic activities of loop diuretics. The combination may cause more acute renal dysfunction than ACE inhibitors alone.

(continues)

Sample Drug Interaction Alerts *(continued)*

Alert No. 2
Interaction: Gabapentin and metronidazole
Severity: Moderate

Effect: The combination of metronidazole and derivatives and ethanol may produce alcohol intolerance reactions. Topically applied, metronidazole would not be expected to produce this reaction based on data indicating lack of absorption. Intravaginal metronidazole may be absorbed and could potentially lead to this reaction.

Note: Alerts were captured from the eRx NOW application, though many other e-prescribing applications use the same or similar content provider for interactions.

The first alert provides specific information on drugs not prescribed and relies on an implicit assumption of a class effect. In addition, the combination of an ACE inhibitor and diuretic is frequently used to manage disease states such as heart failure. More information, such as the patient's current serum creatinine and potassium, is needed. In fact, that information is needed regardless of the presence of an interaction due to the nature of the drugs themselves.

The second alert identifies gabapentin as related to ethanol and from there generalizes to the interaction between metronidazole and ethanol. The alert has no sensitivity to the form of metronidazole prescribed and generates an alert irrelevant to this prescription for topical lotion. Also, how should the severity rating of moderate be interpreted? Antacids can bind with gabapentin and cause a loss of up to 20% of the dose, decreasing the effectiveness of therapy. This is also a moderate severity reaction.

Prescribers do pay attention to interaction alerts more than other alert types,[64] and interaction alerts do provide a safety benefit; however, the examples underscore the need to further develop interaction alerts and provide more robust controls.[100,102]

Emerging Features

Unlike the basic functions and clinical alert checking that already have a widespread presence, the following are clinical decision support features emerging in various applications.

- *Therapy Alerts*: ⊕ Therapy alerts, as opposed to drug alerts, are based on a patient's diagnosis, drug prescribed, laboratory data, medication history, adherence patterns, and patient demographics to provide information relevant to the therapy under consideration.[71] The value of therapy alerts provides an incentive for attaching a diagnosis to the prescription during ordering and for keeping a current problem list in the e-prescribing application. An example of this alert could be a warning that naproxen or pseudoephedrine might be bad for the patient's high blood pressure. If the patient didn't have high blood pressure, this alert wouldn't display. Therapy alerts may also identify drugs that might be treating the side effect of another drug. For example, a warning may suggest an antihistamine with strong anticholinergic properties isn't a good choice for the Alzheimer's patient receiving a medication that enhances cholinergic effects.

- *Setting Alert Display States*: ⊕ The ability to set alerts to an active or passive state is an important feature to limit alert fatigue.[64] Passive alerts are unobtrusively available if the prescriber desires, while active alerts interrupt the prescribing process and force prescriber action. Current implementations of this feature allow global changes to be made—an all-or-none approach. Future refinements may include the ability to customize alerts on an individual alert level and/or patient-specific level.

- *Therapy Dose Limits*: ⊕ Refined upper and lower dose limits based on the patient's diagnosis and age extend the simple drug dosing checks into the clinically relevant therapy dose checks. An example of this alert might be a warning that points out the prescribed dose of levodopa/carbidopa for restless legs syndrome is too high, although it's within the acceptable limits for a patient with Parkinson's disease.

- *Adherence Alerts*: ⊕ Adherence alerts combine prescription refill history, claims data for healthcare visits, and laboratory results to assist prescribers in the formation of specific questions for the patient visit. For example, if the cardiologist was seen as scheduled, the prescriber may order a medication change based on the cardiologist's recommendations. If the cardiologist visit was missed, perhaps delaying a change in medication therapy until the visit can be made is more appropriate. Regardless of the specific situation, the information from adherence alerts can support a decision to increase a dose or keep the same regimen.

Testing Tip

To test the application's dose checking ability, one could try prescribing 8 grams of acetaminophen, 125 mg of digoxin, and diltiazem CD 120 mg three times daily. Respectively, these three orders test OTC dose checking, decimal errors, and frequency errors. Some applications are starting to build intelligence that shows promise, though most lack the robustness necessary to support widespread adoption.

- *Pediatric Dosing Alerts*: ⊕ These alerts are similar to the upper and lower limits but involve more calculations and information. An e-prescribing application should have a field for weight and height to support these calculations. Some specialized applications do a great job with pediatric dose calculations and dosage checks, but the feature hasn't reached mainstream as yet.

Potential Enhancements for CDS

There is a large gap between the CDS available and what CDS could be, and the gap is shrinking every day. This section discusses the features that fill that gap, some of which are available in at least one application and others that may be several years in the future. Demand drives supply. One who sees a feature particularly relevant to one's practice should point it out to the vendor and explain how it would help. Enhancement requests influence the priorities for e-prescribing application vendors.

Configurations and Controls

Alerts are a staple tool for CDS, but more robust controls are needed to combat alert fatigue. The user should be able to:

- Suppress a particular alert for a particular patient for a specified time period and user.[103,104] If the drug interaction is intentional (as is the case with some HIV drug combinations), there is no need to constantly view an alert for a known and intentional interaction in that patient. Drugs such as warfarin are titrated to effect, accounting for the presence of chronic interacting medications that are at times unavoidable. Selective suppression is a useful tool to maximize the number of clinically significant alerts that trigger when working with a patient's information. Suppression shouldn't turn off the alert entirely; just make it inconspicuous for a period of time. Finally, the ability to provide alert suppression for an individual user allows the alert to display (for safety reasons) to other users who may not be familiar with the interaction.

- Suppress an alert for a diagnosis or condition. Clinicians intimately familiar with the effects of medications on a condition they treat frequently may find many of the drug/disease alerts unnecessary.[64] Rather than disabling all drug/disease alerts, suppression of alerts in a particular diagnosis or condition decreases the potential for alert fatigue and, by extension, the potential for error. The same controls mentioned previously are needed: a time limit for the suppression and suppression at a user level.

- Choose between mixed active and passive settings. Active alerts halt the flow of prescribing while passive alerts do not. Globally, interaction alerts of the highest severity could be set to display actively while interactions that are moderately severe or lower are shown passively. This flexibility in display may increase the clinical relevance of the information shown while preserving accessibility of more detailed alert information.[104]

- Designate the timing of alerts. The usual procedure of accepting an order and then seeing an alert is inefficient. The alert needs to display prior to advancing down the path of order entry. Controls that allow the user to determine whether the alert displays retroactively or proactively are needed.[73]

Proactive Alerts

One example of proactive alerts is seen in the eRx NOW application. Interacting drugs are highlighted in the selection list and a hover tip providing more detail about the interaction appears when the cursor is moved above the interacting drug. All this happens in a passive fashion before the drug is chosen, allowing the prescriber to experience fewer alerts as a result of choosing drugs without alert flags. See Figure 4.2 for an example of medication selection.

- Separate alerts by type. Alerts fall into the following two broad categories: clinical and formulary. This subdivision helps to reduce alert fatigue when the prescriber can choose how to address the alerts generated, especially when combined with the passive/active option. The combination provides just-in-time information depending on the specific situation and the familiarity of the prescriber with the drug. Familiar or expected alerts can be passed over for the more unfamiliar and serious alerts.

Having the ability to adjust and configure alerts is critical to avoiding alert fatigue. Patient safety is enhanced when providers can view timely, relevant information at the point of prescribing.[58,64,76,99,100]

 Testing Tip

When evaluating an existing or future e-prescribing application, the user should consider testing it with the following practical examples:

(continues)

Testing Tip *(continued)*

• **What is captured?**

  • Warfarin daily with sertraline 25 mg daily. (Delayed effect, moderate interaction, fair documentation.)

  • Levothyroxine daily and calcium supplements. (The tester should ask whether interactions with OTC medications are captured.)

  • Warfarin daily with alfalfa. (Delayed effect, minor interaction, fair documentation. The tester should ask whether interactions with supplements are captured.)

• **What can be done with the alerts?** Warfarin daily and aspirin 81 mg. (Delayed effect, major interaction, excellent documentation.) Without getting into the patient populations for whom this combination is appropriate, the user should determine whether this interaction can be suppressed without losing the ability to capture other major interactions.

• **Are alerts differentiated?** The evaluator should test formulary alerts by prescribing a brand name for which there is a known generic. Some examples are Glucophage (metformin), Celexa (citalopram), and Norvasc (amlodipine). Then evaluators should try prescribing a brand for which there is a generic available in a different drug class such as Nexium (omeprazole) or any angiotensin II receptor blocker (ARB)/angiotensin converting enzyme inhibitor (ACEI). The evaluator should note whether formulary alerts appear the same as or different from clinical alerts.

Dose Limits

Better decisions can be made when dose limits can draw on information such as diagnosis or laboratory results in the integrated application that is often lacking in the stand-alone e-prescribing application.[91] If the diagnosis, frequently driven by ICD-9 codes, isn't available from the e-prescribing application directly, integration with other healthcare systems can supply it. That, combined with lab data, delivers the information needed to create more refined dosing alerts.

Diagnosis Limits

Ropinirole 9 mg three times daily may be appropriate for Parkinson's disease, but it is a relative overdose if the intent is to treat restless legs syndrome. Likewise, ropinirole 0.25 mg once daily is a relative underdose for treating Parkinson's.

Renal and Hepatic Limits

Ciprofloxacin 500 mg twice daily should generate an alert if the patient has a serum creatinine of 2.5 mg/dL. Incorporating significant laboratory results into the checking process gives greater flexibility to dose limits that are more appropriate for the patient's condition.

Frequency Limits

Lisinopril six times daily should be questioned. Sustained-release anything more than three times daily should likewise be investigated. Dosing alerts should have usual frequency of administration incorporated into their logic.

Duration Limits

Some drug interactions are more problematic in chronic, daily administration as opposed to PRN (as needed) administration. Sumatriptan and sertraline both increase the risk of serotonin syndrome, yet sumatriptan is taken as needed for migraines while sertraline is taken every day for depression (among other indications). Tramadol, used for pain relief, also increases serotonin levels. Based on duration, prescribing tramadol three times daily for 2 weeks in a patient taking sertraline should generate a stronger alert than prescribing sumatriptan as needed. For example, the tramadol triggers an active alert while the sumatriptan alert is displayed passively.

To summarize, the dose alerts should be patient specific, accounting for diagnosis, frequency, duration, and renal/hepatic function. The one-size-fits-all approach generates alert fatigue. The interaction of aspirin 81 mg and warfarin should be in a different category of interaction than aspirin 650 mg four times daily and warfarin. The next generation of alerts need to reflect that difference.[99]

Proactive Dietary Supplement Guidance

Dietary supplements are a billion-dollar industry. Chances are very good that patients take dietary supplements, and dietary supplements interact with drugs. Unfortunately, patients tend not to report supplement use when asked.

Patients have very different definitions of the words *supplement, herbal,* and *vitamin.* For many, the doctor's office handles medicine while the experts on supplements are their friends, nutrition store clerks, the internet, and popular books. The message of natural and safe is so deeply embedded in supplement marketing that it skews perceptions when a healthcare provider asks about supplement use.

⊕ **E-prescribing has the opportunity to provide a very specific tool to assist in drawing out supplement use from patients.** The current applications include supplement interaction checking. However, the application gains additional value when it provides specific prompts to determine supplement use.

Patients use supplements as a form of self-treatment. It follows that the condition that drew the patient to the medical office is probably not one he or she is self-treating—at least not successfully. What are the most likely supplements the patient uses? That depends on the patient's associated comorbidities. For instance, a high proportion of diabetic patients also suffer from depression. It is possible that they come to the office for their insulin prescription but use St. John's wort to self-treat depression.

Using this logic, the e-prescribing application could present the prescriber with likely dietary supplements based on the patient's active problem list and common comorbid conditions. Asking targeted questions about supplements is one way to ensure the medication profile is as accurate as possible. With the list provided by the e-prescribing application, the prescriber knows what questions to ask. Ideally, the list is filtered to contain the supplements that represent the greatest risk either from a disease/supplement interaction or a drug/supplement interaction.

A common question patients ask is, "Can I take this with my other medications?" The e-prescribing application is in a position to provide an answer. The sister to the list of likely supplements is the list of supplements the patient should specifically avoid. For example, high-dose vitamin E or supplements rich in vitamin K should be avoided in the patient on warfarin; St. John's wort and antidepressants don't mix.

Cotherapy Guidance

⊕ **Many medications are monitored with specific tests, and a reminder of that test, when prescribing, is helpful.**[91,105] For example, hydroxychloroquine should trigger the reminder for regular eye exams. New orders for lipid-lowering agents should prompt a review of a fasting lipid profile. Running these alerts through the HIE's data may identify if the eye exam or lab test was done, decreasing alert fatigue.

⊕ **The suggestion of co-ordered drugs at the point of prescribing or just after accepting an order has the potential to make prescribing more efficient and appropriate.** Many therapies are (or should be) ordered with other agents. For example: furosemide and potassium, opiates and stool softeners, bisphosphonates and calcium should be ordered together. This feature is best implemented by applications that support bundling of orders together.

Drug/Lab and Drug/Disease Alerts

Higher levels of integration between applications allow the comparison of diagnoses and lab results with prescription data to make this alert flag available. In this environment, the danger of prescribing a drug with defined contraindications can be communicated to the prescriber. For example:

- *Drug/Lab Contraindication*: The application alerts the prescriber of an elevated potassium level when prescribing an ACEI, a medication that can increase potassium.

- *Drug/Disease Contraindication*: The application alerts the prescriber of the patient's diagnosis of bulimia when prescribing buproprion, a medication that should be avoided in bulimics.

Pharmacist Perspective

Pharmacy applications perform clinical alert checking. E-prescribing applications perform clinical alert checking. Integrated applications perform clinical alert checking. As clinical decision support matures, the clinical alert functions may migrate to a higher, integrated level to reduce redundancy. Like the current subscription to drug databases, the clinical alerts may be processed at an HIE level and fed back to the pharmacy or e-prescribing application.

Patient Demographic Alerts

Patient demographics are underrepresented in the field of CDS alerts.

 A patient's gender, pregnancy, breastfeeding status, age, race, religion, and address are all components that should be taken into account when writing a prescription. Some applications will provide clinical alert checking on a few conditions, but no application covers all of them. As mentioned previously, alerts need to be patient specific. For example, some applications supply a global pregnancy alert during prescribing regardless of the patient's actual pregnancy status or gender. The following are examples of demographic-based alerts.

Gender: Few medications have specific contraindications based solely on gender, though certain alerts are certainly worth heeding. This alert has a quality assurance role. If the wrong patient is chosen, a mismatch between gender and gender-specific drug can alert the prescriber of the error. See also Chapter 9.

Testing Tip

An application evaluator can enter the following orders to test for this type of safety check: estring (estradiol vaginal ring) for a man and alprostadil injection for a woman. The evaluator should note whether there are any alerts.

Pregnancy/Breastfeeding Status: This alert is especially valuable when applied retroactively to a patient's medical profile, such as when a patient is surprised by pregnancy. In that scenario, alerts quickly identify problematic medications and suggest safer alternatives. The more information captured by the application, the more useful this alert can be. The program should support the entry of a due date and it should have the option to automatically apply breastfeeding status for 6 months after the due date. The evaluator should check whether trimesters are indicated or used in the alerts.

 Testing Tip

To test the e-prescribing application for this alert, the evaluator can enter lisinopril 10 mg daily or warfarin 5 mg daily in a profile that identifies the patient as pregnant. To test breastfeeding alerts, he or she can enter an order for methotrexate 7.5 mg weekly or an order for a nicotine patch and then make note of any alerts.

Age: Both pediatric dosing alerts and geriatric alerts are needed. Initial drug doses that are appropriate when a patient is 40 years old are not appropriate at 80 years old. The body changes as we age, accumulating more fat and losing lean muscle mass. Drug distribution changes, metabolism shifts, and kidney function declines. Age-based alerts are needed to reduce the initial doses and avoid medications known to be problematic in the elderly, such as those on the Beers list.

Finding the Beers List

Information on the Beers list can be found at these web sites:[106,107]

Duke University Center for Clinical and Genetic Economics: The Beers list with links to drug information and the original article. www.dcri.duke .edu/ccge/curtis/beers.html

(continues)

Finding the Beers List *(continued)*

Texas Association of Homes and Services for the Aging: The Beers list with explanations about the hazards and relative severity of selected medications in the elderly. www.tahsa.org/files%2FDDF%2Fmedbeer1.pdf

---

Just-in-time information may improve prescribing for the elderly by displaying the relative benefit of prophylactic medications. A daily aspirin prevents cardiovascular events such as a heart attack or stroke, but how much time is needed for the beneficial effect to appear? Will the 93-year-old see the benefit in the remaining years of her life? Until technology matures to support more complex evaluations, a simple trigger based on the patient's age for select medications may be helpful.

 Testing Tip

The evaluator can enter an order for propoxyphene 65 mg on an 85-year-old patient. An alert should appear if comprehensive age-based alerts are present. Propoxyphene is on the Beers list.

Race: Certain medications display race-selective effectiveness. Alerts sensitive to these situations provide a much needed level of patient specificity.

 Testing Tip

The combination of hydralazine and nitrates is reported to be particularly effective for heart failure in African Americans. The tester can enter an order for sustained-release isosorbide mononitrate 60 mg daily and hydralazine 25 mg four times daily in a patient's profile once with African American descent indicated and once for a patient with a different race indicated. The application should provide clinical efficacy information related to the drug selection for each choice.

Religion: Certain religions affect therapies in unanticipated ways. Prescribers need to know whether a Jehovah's Witness patient can receive factor VIII therapy and whether a Muslim can receive porcine-based heparin. They must also know about the religious beliefs concerning human insulin and other biologic drugs. Incorporating religion-driven alerts can help to avoid inflicting ethical and moral dilemmas on patients.

Testing Tip

The tester can enter an order for intravenous immune globulin for a Jehovah's Witness patient. Immune globulin is derived from blood and plasma donations. The tester should note whether any alerts appeared.

Address: A patient's address is a subtle factor in prescribing that can be an invisible source of error. Some medications require a specialty pharmacy to compound and deliver. Therapies for home infusion are particularly affected. Without an appreciation for the patient's physical location, a therapy may be delayed and cause significant harm to the patient. For example, a prescriber orders intravenous antibiotics to be started on a patient living in a remote area during the winter. The pharmacy compounds and delivers the medication 6 hours later, at which point the home-care nurse discovers intravenous access is lost. The need for additional supplies and orders further delays the therapy and hospitalization is required. Having a reminder, even if passive, when ordering time-sensitive medications for patients more than 20 miles from the pharmacy or medical office may be helpful.

Hopefully, future applications will appreciate the contributions patient demographics can make to clinical decision support. Further work is needed to bind the pieces of information together in a meaningful way. Prescribers should work with their e-prescribing vendors to incorporate those alerts most useful to their practice.

Integrated Documentation

How will others know and understand why an alert was overridden, or whether a different agent was chosen because of an alert? In the integrated healthcare application, users in different locations may not have access to the same level of CDS. The medication prescribed at the primary care physician's office is displayed to the cardiologist through the HIE, but there's no documentation of the rationale as to why that particular agent was chosen. Integrated documentation provides that explanation.

The prescriber needs to document the reason an alert was bypassed. The prescription for amoxicillin in the patient with a penicillin allergy could have been an error or intentional. Perhaps the patient only experiences an upset stomach. Or maybe it's just a rash and the prescriber also ordered an antihistamine along with the amoxicillin.

Other circumstances occur in which documentation of adverse effects and therapy success is needed. E-prescribing has the potential to capture this information, but widespread implementation is lacking.

Integrated Resources

Many e-prescribing applications link other tools and resources to provide value-added functions.[108] These functional partnerships may result in embedded web search tools, dosing calculators, context-sensitive drug information, and more. The larger HIE-based health information exchanges frequently use this strategy to bring together useful clinical functions. EMRs and other healthcare applications may also provide this functionality.

A good understanding of the vendor's partnerships helps when the tester is troubleshooting issues regarding embedded mini-applications. The evaluator must know if a vendor partner released a new version of its mini-application that isn't compatible with the e-prescribing application. Likewise, the evaluator should know if the vendor partner's mini-application is upgraded when new versions are available, or whether the vendor applies upgrades.

Example

An e-prescribing application links to a dosing calculator supplied by partner *X*, which has just been bought by another company. How will this affect the user's experience the next time the dose calculator is used? How long will support for the dose calculator be provided?

Implementation of Standards

Certification that an application meets a standard does not mean the implementation of the standard is appropriate. Evaluators should always test prospective e-prescribing applications for usability. The context and workflow the application operates within is critical to the relative safety of the overall process.

The ability to enter a patient's allergy is nearly worthless if the feature is poorly documented and buried beneath a 12-step process.

Pharmacist Perspective

A pharmacy-specific example of this implementation is the display of the physician comments within the pharmacy program. The evaluator should ask the following questions: Are physician comments prominently displayed as

(continues)

Pharmacist Perspective *(continued)*

an alert? Are they passively accessible during order entry? Do they require users to travel to another portion of the program and actively search for the comments? Many systems claim to uphold the standard of making prescriber comments available, but which system is safest and easiest to use?

The safety implications of poorly implemented standards are serious. The standard may be supporting safety features that become turned off or bypassed in favor of a more efficient workflow. Adoption of e-prescribing technology may be delayed as the application fails to meet user expectations. Standards are important, but just as important is the way the standards are applied to serve the prescriber's workflow and the safety of the patient.[109]

Designer Details

Application designers should involve tech-savvy, working clinicians in all stages of product development, not just during final product testing.

Conclusion

Attention to the larger picture by vendors and RHIOs is needed to create systems that work together to promote safety across the spectrum of use. No longer can an application be conceived to merely fulfill a role in a contained and isolated office. Developing advanced clinical decision support requires more intensive information resources. The changes sweeping through health care have the potential to gather the functions of isolated applications and knit them into a safety net for the patient.[90]

To accomplish this goal, the industry needs to hear the voice of the clinicians. These clinicians should tell their vendors what is needed, not just what is convenient or easy. What will make the care given patients safer and better? Maintaining a patient-centric approach, delivered through office-centric workflows, is essential for driving utility into the applications we use on a daily basis.

Chapter 8

Evaluating E-Prescribing Applications

Prescribers . . . . Required
Nurse/medical assistants . . . . Suggested
Office managers . . . . Required
Pharmacists . . . . Suggested
E-Rx application designers . . . . Required

Choosing an e-prescribing application for a medical practice is a complex affair that involves clinical, financial, and regulatory interests. Sometimes the choice is already made and a clinician is asked to comment on the application's use in the clinical setting. This chapter discusses clinical aspects of e-prescribing with a special focus on features related to patient safety. For the sake of illustration, eRx NOW screen shots are used, though the discussion is not limited to eRx NOW or its functions. We'll progress from user-interface issues and proceed through a typical prescription workflow. Questions are presented to help guide an assessment or evaluation of the e-prescribing application. The details behind many of these questions can be found in other chapters but are presented here in a consolidated form for easy reference. Those who have access to a working application should consider using the testing tips in Appendix C to round out an evaluation.

User Interface Considerations

The application's user interface is an important, though often underestimated, safety feature. In many cases, the person choosing or evaluating the

---

E-Rx Example

To see the eRx NOW application in action, consider reviewing the tutorials available by clicking on the Help icon at http://erxnow.allscripts.com. The application provides a frame of reference for subsequent discussions; the tutorials walk through many features common to electronic prescribing applications. The purpose of our discussion is to generalize from these common features and apply the concepts to other e-prescribing applications.

---

application has a familiarity with computers and technology that is not shared by many of the staff who will ultimately be using the application. When performing an evaluation, always consider the perspective of each role that interacts with the application, including the secretary, office manager, nurse, and prescriber.

• Who are the primary users of the e-prescribing application? What is their familiarity with computers?

Log-In

The first interaction a user has with the application is the log-in screen, as **Figure 8.1** shows. The important feature is the lack of features. Unlike some web pages where a log-in is buried in a corner or tucked away in a sidebar, the log-in is prominently displayed. Those who wish to view interactive tutorials can click the help icon (in eRx NOW, the help icon is the question mark) and select the tutorials option on the resulting page.

From a safety perspective, this page demonstrates two key principles—simplicity and redundancy. The simplicity of the page draws attention to the log-in and user name fields. Options other than the user name and password fields are displayed as icons with a minimum of text. In fact, the hyperlinks in the text lead to the same places as the icons, underscoring the redundancy of navigation methods.

Different people learn in different ways. Providing more than one way to access a function caters to these different styles. Accomplishing this in the simplest way possible increases the safety in the system. An uncluttered log-in increases the likelihood that a user can successfully log in. If the log-in was less intuitive, the chances of the application being used are correspondingly lower.[18] The evaluator should consider whether it is easy enough for someone to sign in while talking on the phone. The information in the e-prescribing application may be crucial to the conversation, but if the log-in is frustrating, the easier choice may be to write down notes and call back later, if there is an opportunity later.

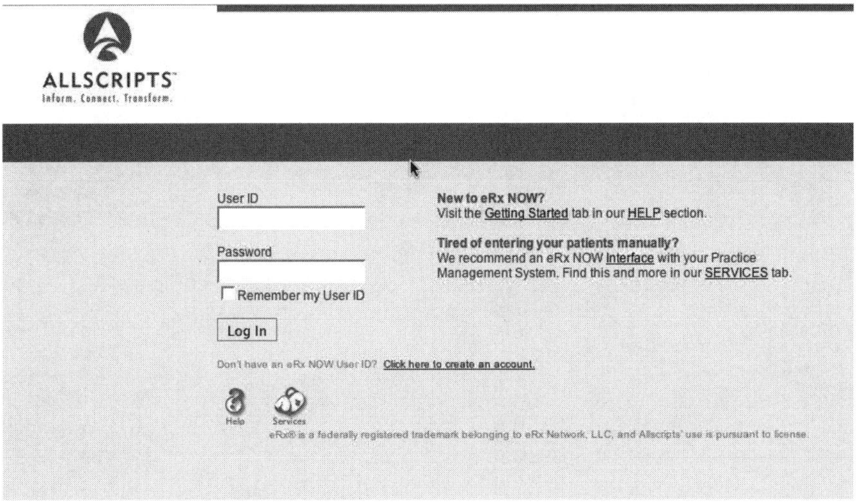

FIGURE 8.1 eRx NOW Log-In
Source: Copyright 2007 Allscripts.

Integrated systems remove this step entirely through single sign-on technology, or SSO technology. The integrated application (an EMR, healthcare portal, or clinical system) passes the user name and password to the e-prescribing application. The result is one fewer step and less potential for error.

• How intuitive is the log-in process?

• Does the user receive help or promptings when incorrect passwords or user names are entered? Could a part-time employee returning from an extended leave log on without difficulty?

Layout

Once someone is logged in, the eRx NOW application displays a patient search screen.

In the integrated application, patient context may be passed between applications. A patient who is selected and active in the EMR or practice management system will be the same patient accessed in the e-prescribing application. A stand-alone application displays a blank page without any patient selected.

Figure 8.2 displays the patient search page for an assistant view. The view would be different if a prescriber logged in, which highlights another important safety feature: the ability to alter the user interface

ALLSCRIPTS

Patient:	[No Patient Selected]	Gender, DOB:		MRN:		KMMC Family Practice
Active allergies:						Nurse GRIPA
Active problems:						
Active medications:						
Pharmacy:						

Help Services Profile Log Out

Patients | Tasks (8) | Reports | Settings

Google Custom Search
Search

Choose Patient: test   [Search] [Add Patient]

Help With This Screen

[Check In] [Renew] [Review History] [Select Provider ▼] [New Rx]

Important Information

MRN⇕	Patient Name⇕	DOB	SSN	Phone Number	Street Address
8888	Allscripts, Test	05/25/1965	123-45-6789		222 Main Street
127638	Downieville, Test	06/01/1970	882-76-5589		4321 Main Street
987654	HCP, Test	12/21/1979	555-33-4444		222 Main Street
12345	HealthCare Partners, Test	06/01/1943	999-88-7777		222 Main Street
AHS274	Hoag, Test	12/12/1976			1234 Main Street
77889	IMMC, Test	02/23/1977	987-65-4321		1212 Main Street
AHS216	Loso, Test	09/10/1982		802-434-5345	20 Lawrence Rd
AHS248	Mark, Test	09/09/2001			
AHS186	Mickey, Test	09/08/1965			5000 Fairway Drive
AHS275	Newport Beach, Test	03/16/1970			555 Tiffany Drive
AHS72	O'Neil, Test	04/09/1955		847-909-4539	
AHS276	Orange County, Test	12/26/1941			One Sherwood Drive
AHS246	Patient Ntsp, Test	01/01/1980		512-633-6515	
AHS288	Patient, Test	03/03/1981		708-485-1424	
AHS289	Patient, Test	03/03/1929		847-234-7260	
TESTMRN	Patient, Test	09/14/1967	999-99-9999	585-2355867	2800 Harris Street
AHS257	Patient, Test	09/08/1954			
AHS241	Patient, Test	08/18/1984			
AHS234	Patient, Test	07/19/1954			
AHS226	Patient, Test M	12/12/2000			
AHS156	Patient, Test Y	05/24/2007			

Page 1 [2] [3]

FIGURE 8.2 Patient Search
Source: Copyright 2007 Allscripts.

based on designated role. From a safety perspective, this drives a number of other significant features that would not be possible otherwise.

The color scheme is simple, consistent, and does not distract from important elements. Jarring color schemes draw attention to noncritical areas; this works against the user the way water wears away stone. Without an interface that is comfortable to navigate, the potential for error increases.[72]

Spacing is sufficient to display the information without mashing lines together. Adequate margins are important. Clumping small text together makes for difficult reading and increases the potential for error,[72] especially when making selections from a narrow, crowded list.

Finding the right patient is made easier through the use of smart searching. The user should try using the first three letters or numbers of a patient's first name, last name, phone number, address, or Social Security number, or combination thereof to generate a list of matches.

Interactive areas are clearly and intuitively labeled with fonts that are easy to read. Users would be confused if a programmer decided to label the Patients tab as entities, recipients, clients, customers, supplicants, primary records, people, humans, or subjects. Proper labeling is essential for the users of the application who bring along preconceived

Designer Details

The use of color as the sole identifier of difference should be avoided; some users are color blind. Color may be used to supplement differentiation of **application elements** but should never be used as the sole means of differentiation. The designer should consider alternatives such as shape or location instead.

definitions of what terms mean. When a mismatch occurs between the user's expectation and the programmer's intention, the potential for error increases.

• Can you easily recognize application functions such as medication history and medication renewals?

• Can you easily recognize application content such as patient demographics and medication orders?

Consistent placement of the interactive and static areas makes the application easier to learn. In eRx NOW, the patient's information stays at the top the screen throughout the prescription-writing process. As users learn the application, their eyes track to areas containing the information. When layouts shift from screen to screen, the potential for error increases.

A feature not seen in this application is pop-up windows. The proliferation of windows is disruptive to the interface as evidenced by a pop-up blocker feature on most web browsers. It is easy to lose one's place in the multitude of windows present on the screen. This draws energy and focus away from the critical task of managing a patient's prescriptions.

• Does the program follow normal computer conventions for actions? Do the buttons, links, and menus perform expected functions?

• Are labels for buttons and key areas of the program labeled in a meaningful way for a clinician? Are there elements with labels that appear unclear?

Support for Different Roles

Prescribers and staff perform different functions and have different responsibilities in the prescribing process. In general, prescribers generate and approve prescriptions while staff manage renewals and patient demographics. The most efficient presentation displays only those elements the user needs. Dividing the user interface into two separate presentations based on functional role allows the exclusion of features that would otherwise contribute to screen clutter and confusion. As a result of this specialization, the assistant view prominently displays functions not visible to the prescriber, and the prescriber's view prominently displays functions not visible to the assistant. Each view is customized to the needs of the user.

The eRx NOW application makes a small modification depending on whether the user is an administrator or not. Administrators have the settings tab visible, whereas users do not. Visually removing elements that are not accessible or not relevant enhances the overall safety of the application.

The division of roles between users and administrators provides security advantages as well. Local control over users expands the options for troubleshooting without the need to go through telephonic help or wait for a contracted agency to come.

Change Control

Local control provides flexibility. When staffing levels change due to sick calls or vacations, appropriate role-based functions can be added to an individual's profile. User profiles for temporary or transient help can be added and removed easily. Contrast this with a centralized governance model where administrative control is managed remotely and turnaround time can be lengthy.

Role Support Enhancements

What could be done to improve on the foundation of role division? The function can be expanded and pushed much further. Having roles that reflect the diversity of practices and professions in the community is a good start.

For example, physician assistants in New York have specific requirements surrounding prescribing. In the outpatient setting, they must have the name of the covering physician's name appear on the prescription. Medical residents in New York also need to have the name of the attending physician appear on the prescription to allow pharmacies to correctly bill certain insurances. The two roles of assistant and prescriber are not sufficient to capture the needs of different types of prescribers; more role types are needed.

In addition to different types of prescribers, the application should accommodate different types of assistants as well; medical assistants, medical secretaries, office managers, licensed practical nurses, registered nurses, medical students, and pharmacists all have responsibilities within the prescriptive process.

Designer Details

A flexible interface is desirable, but not at the cost of complexity. Application designers should consider providing predefined user profiles to facilitate setup. Rather than requiring the administrator to adjust every setting such as disallowing schedule II prescriptions for the physician assistant, the designer could allow the selection of the type of user from the outset, and the selection would contain the preset configuration. Finer adjustments can easily be made afterwards to account for state-specific regulations.

During the initial user setup, designers should consider adding on-screen explanations of what the option allows or disallows with a specific case example where possible. For instance, if the DEA schedule II box is checked, does that mean schedule II (C-II) prescriptions can or cannot be prescribed? Clarity is needed for the administrators who are often clinicians or office managers.

• Does the application support role-based interfaces?

• How robust are the roles in the e-prescribing application? Can a nurse, physician assistant, medical resident, nurse practitioner, and physician be assigned functions for processing prescriptions that accommodate workflows and state laws?

Accessibility

Features are generally no more than one to two mouse clicks away through the use of a tabbed interface and hyperlinks, demonstrating good accessibility. The steps needed to complete a process are minimized with the result that workflow is enhanced. This horizontal presentation, as opposed to a vertical presentation, makes finding relevant information and features efficient. Redundancy is built into the interface, further increasing the exposure of key areas to the user. For example, the user can click the edit allergies hyperlink to access the allergies page or select a button within the patient edit screen that takes him or her to the same place.

• Are there forcing functions that promote safety such as context-sensitive buttons and menus?

Cross-Platform Consistency

The e-prescribing application's interface needs to be consistent across other areas of computing, such as the internet, cell phones, traditional desktop computers, laptops, PDAs, and tablet

computers for the reasons we've been discussing. When features and functions vary depending on the device used to interact with the application, confusion and the potential for error ensue. This means the presentation should be consistent, functions should be accessible, and the user interface should approximate the standard application interface to the greatest degree possible.

 Testing Tip

When evaluating an e-prescribing application supported by multiple devices, the tester should perform the following actions on each device: enter a patient, enter an allergy, enter a new prescription, send the prescription to a pharmacy, send the prescription to a printer, renew a prescription, and resolve a clinical alert. This series of tests covers most areas of variations encountered between devices.

• Is the application's interface consistent across platforms?

Mouse and Key Enhancements

Constantly switching between a keyboard and mouse interrupts efficient workflow. Both modes of work should be supported to the fullest extent possible. The reasons for this are twofold: efficiency and disaster planning. Disruptions to the normal workflow increase the potential for error. In general, the greater the disruption, the greater the potential for error.

If an e-prescribing application requires the presence of both a mouse and a keyboard, the loss of either component results in a total loss of functionality. If the application can be fully operated by either input device, the loss of one does not prevent the application from being used, and workflow is disrupted to a lesser extent.

As easy as a computer mouse (or equivalent pointing device) is for learning and demonstration, e-prescribing applications need to function fully in the absence of a mouse for optimal efficiency. An application that can be run by keyboard only will outpace a mouse-driven application on most days. Unfortunately, the learning curve for keyboard commands is steeper. Even so, the ability to drive the application entirely from the keyboard allows users to migrate from the mouse to the keyboard as familiarity with the application increases. Some keyboard enhancements to look for are:

• *Keyboard Shortcuts:* Can the application's functions be called up with specific key combinations? Are those combinations visible in contextual help menus?

- *Short Codes:* Can the application support user-defined short codes for common orders and actions? For example, could LIS10D call up the order for lisinopril 10 mg tablets, take one tablet daily, dispense no. 30, refill ×12? Appropriately implemented (there are certainly risks that need to be controlled), short codes can greatly speed order entry.

- *Character Filtering:* Entry is made faster when the list of choices narrows with every character entered into the search field. Rather than adding a test phrase and clicking a button to send the query, results are displayed as the user types.

Short Codes

Using short codes may cause more problems than it solves in applications without appropriate safeguards to prevent wrong-order entry. The potential for error increases with the degree of complexity of the short codes. At a minimum, verification of the short code results should be included as a forcing function. For example, if LIS10D retrieves lisinopril 10 mg daily, the user needs to confirm that it is the correct order.

The other extreme is full mouse operability. Can the application be operated in the absence of a keyboard? Some mouse enhancements to look for are:

- *Soft-Text Entry:* Does the application have a soft-text input that can be driven by a mouse? Can a virtual keyboard be summoned for quick letter entry? Are single- and multi-letter entries possible?

- *Rapid Browsing:* Does the application support alternative, mouse-driven search strategies such as dynamic filters? For example, can the list of possible patients be narrowed if the mouse is used to choose parameters such as male patients older than 80 years old with heart failure living more than 10 miles from the office?

- *Relational Search Strategies:* Can the application support searching by association? For example: when prescribing, if the prescriber clicks on the patient's active problem of heart failure, does the application display current medications in the patient's profile used to treat the condition as well as a prescribing window with alternative medications?

- *Mouse-Specific Functions:* Is the right mouse button utilized in context-sensitive ways? For example, does right clicking on a patient's name or other identifying information bring up additional navigation and action options such as renewing a medication, creating a new prescription, or adding an allergy?

⚠️ **Incorporating full functionality for both the keyboard and mouse drives efficiency and provides an important safety feature in the event of an emergency.**

• Are the keyboard and mouse controls intuitive? Consistent?

• Are keyboard efficiency enhancements such as shortcuts, short codes, and character filtering available?

• Are mouse efficiency enhancements such as soft-text entry, rapid browsing, relational searching, or context clicking available?

HIE Integration Considerations

Just as the user's interaction with the application affects patient safety, the interaction of other applications with e-prescribing also affects patient safety. An e-prescribing vendor will have to address this higher-level functionality. The application designer will need to consider interface options, add **master patient index (MPI)** resolving ability, and increase the ability of third-party applications to dynamically interact.

⚠️ **A theoretical, futuristic e-prescribing application would accept and send HL-7, CCR, and SCRIPT transactions to accommodate any HIE's needs.** A solid interface with the HIE drives the benefits that higher-level integration allows. Instead of requiring manual data uploads for patient demographics and medication histories, this system supports real-time connections that are easily configured. Resources normally diverted to implement and maintain the relationship with the HIE are returned instead to the office and the patient.

Once an interface is established with the HIE, the next challenge is identifying patients. For example, consider a man named George Brown, who has five sons, all named George. How will integrated applications pull health records on any of these Georges from the lab, hospital, doctor's office, and pharmacy while ensuring that all the records belong to the correct George?

⚠️ **Future e-prescribing applications should include an MPI resolver.**

The MPI provides a way to uniquely identify a given patient. The lab may have a patient's address on Elm Street, while the hospital record shows her living on Parkhurst. Which one is correct? Is it the same patient? Few legacy applications were built with these challenges in mind.

In an ideal e-prescribing application such as the theoretical application mentioned previously, incoming patient records would be matched and merged with the existing records. Records that are close matches would be

Designer Suggestion

Applications should be designed to support both implementation and regular use. Features such as bulk loading and unloading of data facilitate implementation and are useful in other specific-use cases. Once past implementation, the user's focus shifts to the features of regular use. Designers should give consideration to accommodating high-level integration features external to the e-prescribing application that will use the data within the e-prescribing application.

held in a quarantine area for manual resolution. Outbound records would be tagged with a history of prior resolutions to help the receiving system make a match on its end.

Once the HIE received the patient information (indicating the interface is working) and knows it's the correct patient (which would mean the MPI resolver is working), the patient's information could be combined, compared, sorted, and viewed. So how would the ideal e-prescribing application take advantage of the enriched information available at the HIE?

This theoretical e-prescribing application would have a dedicated area that receives patient-specific alerts driven by an external plug-in source such as the HIE.

The plug-in would provide just-in-time information relevant to the prescriber's work.[4] Patient-specific information from labs, community guidelines, and specialty consultations would be combined in a clinically relevant fashion and delivered via a standardized messaging interface, perhaps a secure RDF site summary (RSS) feed. Writing a prescription for lisinopril, a drug eliminated through the kidneys, would trigger a display of the patient's current serum creatinine and potassium as part of the prescribing process. A reminder to check a potassium level in a few weeks would be accessible in the background, along with a link to the last cardiology consultation.

While these features may seem outlandish or impractical, they are actually very close to widespread availability.[110–112] Many organizations are adapting their applications to accomplish similar functions. Even so, to bring the successes of the few into the reach of the many requires further standardization and harmonization of standards.

For example, how will user roles be transferred to integrated systems without standards for security? What standards are in place to manage patient context passing so that integrated systems operate seamlessly with respect to the user? What standards exist to handle the multi-site and multi-organizational configurations required by some healthcare systems?

Much work remains to be done. One of the most important actions a clinician can take is to supply the vendor and HIE with constructive, practical feedback. The resulting changes to the application not only benefit the clinician but also patients and health care in general.

• How does the application manage duplicate patients? Can patients be merged? How are deceased patients managed?

• How compatible is the application with input and output standards such as HL-7, CCR, NCPDP, and X12N? (See also Chapter 2.)

• Does the application support advanced clinical decision support? To what extent? (See also Chapter 7.)

Workflow Considerations

Chapters 3-5 address the elements of e-prescribing in detail. Because workflow is such an important part of e-prescribing, the key questions are presented as a simple list to avoid needless repetition of the previous chapters.

Key Questions for Assistants

• What options are available to enter demographics?

• How are allergies entered? Displayed? How robust are they?

• How are problems and diagnoses entered? Displayed? How robust are they?

• What options are available to enter insurance? Does the program check eligibility?

• What options are available to assign pharmacies to patients? Can users add a pharmacy ad hoc if it isn't available in the selection list?

• Can users print an active patient medication list?

• What sort and view options are available for patients, medication orders, and pharmacies?

• How easy is it to renew medications? Can more than one medication be renewed at a time?

• Are there scheduling or scripting aids for renewals?

Key Questions for Prescribers

Assistant Prescribing Support

Many states allow a nurse or secretary to phone in a prescription for a non-controlled substance on behalf of the prescriber.

- Will nurses have the authority to renew the prescription on behalf of the prescriber in the e-prescribing application?

- Are safeguards needed to prevent a prescription from going to the pharmacy prior to a prescriber's approval?

- What reports are available for monitoring application use and activity? Is there any intelligence within the application to flag suspicious user activity?

- What functions does the e-prescribing application offer supportive prescribing roles?

- Can the e-prescribing application be configured to allow support staff to override some alerts and not others?

- Are favorites, or commonly prescribed medications, supported? How are favorites created?

- Are therapy templates supported, where multiple drugs commonly prescribed together are bundled into a single template?

- How are favorites organized? How are they managed? What maintenance is needed to prune unwanted favorites?

- How easy is medication selection when prescribing? How robust are the search options? How often does the application display the right drug the first time?

- Are custom medication orders supported? Can custom medications orders be saved?

- What filtering is available for medication lists? For past prescriptions? For diagnoses?

- How are patient instructions entered (structured or free form)? Are drop-down lists required? Can complex patient instructions be saved?

- How are formulary alternatives determined? What determines their order when they are displayed? Are there any filters applied, such as drug class?

• Does the application produce legal prescriptions through the printer or fax?

• What medication information is available during prescription generation? What are the sources for the information? The internet? The drug manufacturer?

• How is patient medication information accessed and printed?

Key Administrator Questions

• How intuitive is the management of users? Sites?

• What configuration of sites and practices is available? Can the application accommodate relationships with other practices? What about on-call coverage?

• How are patient demographics loaded? How are patient medication histories loaded?

• Is the e-prescribing application compliant with state laws and regulations?

• Is the e-prescribing application fully supported by infrastructure and product companies? (See also Chapter 2.)

• Does your vendor support optional SCRIPT transactions for cancelling a prescription or allowing a pharmacist to request a change? If not, does the vendor have plans for supporting them? Will that entail a major upgrade?

• What assistant/prescriber interactions are supported? Tasks? Secure communications?

• What reports are available through the e-prescribing application? Can the vendor give a use case example for each report?

• Do the reports meet your needs? Can the format be changed?

• Can users send a patient notification directly from the e-prescribing application? For example, a medication recall or sensational study is released. Can the user send a letter to all patients affected by the news?

• Does the application require monitoring for failed transactions? Does the application have options to automatically resend prescriptions that failed to transmit?

• Does the application capture documentation of therapy effectiveness and reasons for medication discontinuation? Are there other options for documentation in the system?

• How are drug samples handled? How is drug administration in the office handled?

• Are there quizzes, interactive training modules, practical exercises that use the application, or a skill-based evaluation?

• Is computer-based training available? Is a workbook with exercises and examples available as a training aid? Will someone come in and provide a presentation and lecture?

• What training support materials are available? Is retraining available? For how long? Is there a fee?

Advanced Function Considerations

• *Prescribing Limitations:* Can the prescriber have the option to send a prescription to another prescriber for peer review? This is useful in training situations. Can prescriptions be prepared but not authorized, such as the way a nurse or medical assistant might interact with them? Is a password needed to authorize the prescription?

• *Formatting Options:* Can a nonlegal copy of the prescription be printed for informational purposes? Does the content change, such as adding the covering physician's name, depending on the user's role? Are different formatting options available to address needs, such as a prescriber who practices in multiple states?

• *User Interface Options:* Can specific interface elements be selectively hidden for personnel who have no need of those elements? For example, if the secretary is only accessing patient profiles and has no need to renew medication orders, can the renewal function be hidden?

  The ability to selectively remove access to unused features is a powerful tool to drive relevance and safety into the application. Forcing functions serve as an important safety feature by preventing inadvertent actions.

• *Clinical Decision Support Settings:* Can the application be configured to prevent severe clinical alerts from being overridden without an explanation? Can the user select what action is required to override an alert?

Conclusion

Not all questions are applicable to every situation, nor did this chapter provide a comprehensive list of questions to ask. Evaluators should investigate the features most relevant for their work. Very few vendors can satisfy the majority of features these questions represent, yet their response to many of these questions indicates what kind of partner they will be. In many ways, that is the most important feature of an e-prescribing application.

E-Prescribing Safely

Paper Prescribing Systems

In a 2006 report, the Institute of Medicine targeted paper prescriptions for conversion into e-prescriptions by the year 2010. What is it about paper prescriptions that make them so prone to errors? Why are electronic prescriptions so heavily endorsed?

A prescription is a vehicle of communication. The potential for error increases when the amount of communication is reduced or the quality is poor. Factors that degrade the prescription's ability to communicate are causes of potential error in the prescribing system.

Poor handwriting not only fails to communicate, it can provide misinformation. The illegible prescription jeopardizes the safety of the prescriptive process and can contribute to patient harm.[2,11,41]

Legibility describes the form of communication, but what of content? Here, too, the opportunities for error abound. Examples of unclear content include dangerous abbreviations, vague patient instructions, and questionable formulations. Abbreviations and trailing zeros have been prohibited by the Joint Commission for their ability to miscommunicate.[80] In other case examples, key content of the prescription is simply missing; they have no indication, no dispense quantity, no patient age, no date, or no signature.

Other systems affect paper prescriptions, often in subtle ways. For example, the legal system influences communication in ways unnoticed—until the law is broken. Many states have laws that regulate a prescription's form and content. Failure to meet these requirements results in delays and errors. A prescription's ability to communicate is also limited by its physical dimensions. A prescriber can only write so much on a small square pad. This forces prescribers toward brevity with a corresponding tendency to leave out useful information.

Fragile Forms

As an instrument of communication, paper prescriptions are remarkably fragile and prone to error. Patients can (and do) lose prescriptions. Patients can (and do) alter prescriptions. Faxed prescriptions can be altered by the quality of the machines used to transmit them. Some people pull a document through a fax machine just to hurry it up. The receiving fax prints out words resembling long evening shadows. Also, many documents are loaded face up in copiers with auto-feed abilities, while most fax machines require the documents to be face down. Many times prescriptions are faxed, but the pharmacy only receives a blank sheet.

Increasing the number of subsystems in the prescriptive process increases the potential error for a patient. Every fax machine, secretary, nurse, patient, family member, and pharmacy technician is a subsystem. Paper prescriptions are exposed to a wide range of subsystems in their journey to the pharmacy.

For all the glaring concerns surrounding paper systems, there are some redeeming characteristics. Paper systems are very portable. A prescription can be created with very basic equipment, handed to a patient, mailed, or faxed. The ability to draw—a technique used when prescribing medications intended for application to specific places on the body such as an elbow or knee—can enhance communication beyond mere words.

Safety Benefits of E-Prescribing

It's helpful to frame the safety benefits of e-prescribing before spending time mapping the opportunities for error. Many of these features are discussed in Chapters 3 through 5 of this book, but they are worth repeating here in an abbreviated form. Hopefully, other healthcare professionals will see the value of these practices and adopt them.

 Error-Prone Medications: Some medications are more prone to errors than others. In the outpatient setting, 86.5% of preventable adverse drug events were caused by three drug categories: cardiovascular drugs, analgesics, and hypoglycemic agents.[113] This information can be used to modify the prescribing process for medications that fall into these categories.

 Medication List: Many e-prescribing applications have the ability to print a list of active medications for the patient. Patients should be encouraged to carry a list of their medications with them. This list is invaluable should a patient need emergent hospitalization. Every specialist, pharmacist, and other healthcare provider a patient sees will be delighted to have access to the patient's current medications.

 Pharmacist Perspective

Pharmacists also have the ability to print a list of medications from the patient's profile. They can give the patient a printed list of his active medications to take with him to his next doctor's appointment. If printing the list is cumbersome, pharmacists should work with their pharmacy application vendor to make it more convenient.

 Just-in-Time Information: This clinical decision support function is becoming more available. Drug information can be accessed during the prescribing process. Drug interaction details can be viewed before finishing the prescription. Prescribers can get answers to questions more efficiently. (The quality of those answers is another discussion entirely.)

 Direct Communication: The ability to send prescriptions directly to the pharmacist bypasses many systems that would otherwise increase the potential for error. Illegible prescriptions are nearly eliminated.

Recall Reports: Drug recalls at a patient level, such as the one recently experienced when rofecoxib was withdrawn by Merck[114] are facilitated with an electronic prescribing application. Most applications have the ability to print a report that lists patients for whom a particular drug has been prescribed.

Security: E-prescribing applications decrease the opportunity for fraudulent prescribing by nonprescribers.

 Adherence: Adherence remains a soft benefit until data emerges to provide more evidence. Removing patients as transporters of prescriptions overcomes a number of obstacles that intervene from the time a prescription is written to the time it is presented for filling at the pharmacy. This convenience may result in an increase in adherence. There is data that supports an increase in fulfilled prescriptions after the implementation of e-prescribing, but the link to adherence hasn't been made yet.

 Integration: E-prescribing applications are a critical data source for advanced, integrated healthcare initiatives such as HIE networks.

 Disasters: Prescriptions and medication histories in e-prescribing applications can be reconstituted in the event of a disaster such as Hurricane Katrina.

E-Prescribing Applications

Electronic prescribing may improve patient safety, though assuming all e-prescriptions are safer than paper prescriptions is not accurate. The same principle governing quality in paper systems is at work in electronic applications. A prescriber with poor handwriting will have a greater incidence of error than a prescriber with legible writing (assuming other qualities are equal). A prescriber with a poorly implemented e-prescribing system will expose himself or herself to more potential errors than a prescriber with a well-implemented e-prescribing system.

Electronic prescriptions tend to have fewer errors associated with them, though much of the hard data is the result of pioneering efforts from hospital-based computerized physician order entry systems.[5,17,40] Some studies demonstrated an increase in errors, underscoring that safer does not mean error proof.[4,42,43,115]

If paper is eliminated, then from where do these errors come? Many of the new errors in electronic prescribing are the same as those with paper, they are just clothed in electronic form. Other errors are truly new, growing from the new technology and options afforded by an otherwise improved process.

It is important not to confuse types of error with an increase in error frequency. When the prescription travels from the prescriber's computer directly to the pharmacy's computer in an EDI transaction, the complexity added by the patient, nurse, fax machine, pharmacy technicians, copier, and family members is avoided. E-prescriptions bypass entire systems, and reducing the number of systems is a good thing. Pilot studies demonstrate an impressive number of prescriptions changed as a result of safety features present in e-prescribing systems.[43,56] As an example, the Henry Ford Medical Group, part of the Southeast Michigan ePrescribing Initiative, reports 80,000 prescriptions changed or cancelled due to drug interaction alerts, 6,500 potential allergic reactions, and more than 50,000 prescriptions changed or cancelled due to formulary alerts.[116] The discussion that follows, while describing types of errors associated with e-prescribing in detail, does nothing to diminish the safety of e-prescribing over paper prescriptions.

Imagine a prescription pad with marked areas for the drug name, patient name, dose, in fact, for every element of the prescription. The prescriber fills in the blanks, tears off the prescription, and beneath it is another prescription with similar blanks. But these blanks are arranged differently. The drug name is at the bottom instead of the top. The signature line is along the side instead of the middle. The prescription differs in every respect, and yet the content is identical. Flipping forward in this strange prescription pad, the prescriber sees every page has a different layout and organization, though the content is the same on every page. Let's assume the prescriber memorized the places to put all the information on one prescription blank in this strange pad. This is the equivalent of learning one e-prescribing application.

Here is the first opportunity for error in electronic prescribing applications: the user interface.

User Interface Challenges

You Know What I Mean (Not Really)! The Dangers of Choosing the Wrong Drug

 Selecting the wrong drug in e-prescribing is the equivalent of writing a paper prescription such that the pharmacist mistakes the intended drug for something entirely different. Many e-prescribing applications display search results to the prescriber as an alphabetized list of drugs from which to choose. It is easy to click the wrong drug in the selection window. Some applications have a limited display that cuts off the end of the drug name. This is disastrous for combination drugs such as sulfamethoxazole-trimethoprim, lisinopril-hydrochlorothiazide, and simvastatin-ezetemibe. Unless the prescriber pays careful attention, she might not realize that the single drug she thought she was choosing is actually a combination agent.

The user should look for the presence of horizontal scroll bars in the drug selection window and use them. Horizontal scroll bars indicate that more information is only a click away. Users must be sure to read the complete name of the drug before selecting it.

Warning

If a user sees that drug names are truncated and there are no scroll bars, he should stop using the e-prescribing application and go back to paper prescriptions until the issue is fixed. The potential for error is too great. If the vendor can't fix the issue, the prescriber should look for another vendor.

Drugs displayed in small font, one below the other, represent another hazard. The tendency is to identify the desired drug and look to the right for a list of doses that match. The second half of a drug combination effectively disappears, blending in with the confusing clutter of the full drug name. Anything more than twenty letters long taxes the eyes and dulls the brain. This effect is especially true of applications that list comprehensive formulations of a drug. Consider this text entry: "Enoxaparin hydrochloride/100 mg–ml/injectable solution." The dose field would tell the user this is actually a 60 mg prefilled syringe, though at first glance, the concentration can easily be mistaken as a 100 mg dose.

Testing Tip

Search for aspirin and see how easy it is to find a plain 81 mg tablet. If you see pages of formulations, start exploring easy ways to narrow results.
Some applications allow for partial searching such as "asp 81," which can be a huge time-saver (and an important safety feature). Other systems will search the prescriber's favorites and avoid the complex listing entirely—another safety feature.

Some applications don't allow searching by the chemical name if a brand exists without a generic commercially available. The intent is laudable—to only allow selection of commercially available products. In reality, this frustrates the prescribing process and the prescriber. The results may be the wrong drug or formulation. As an example, searching for isradipine 5 mg when Dynacirc CR 5 mg is desired will return isradipine 5 mg immediate release. This medication is intended for twice-daily dosing as opposed to the once-daily formulation the prescriber anticipated.

Prevention: 🖊 **The user should determine if his e-prescribing application can find drugs based on chemical name.** If not, he should make a request to the vendor to add that functionality and search by brand name where possible. Most e-prescribing applications default to allow generic substitution.

Users should evaluate the layout of the displays. Are lines of text double spaced for easier reading? Can the users rapidly and accurately identify the item they're searching for in a list of results? If not, they should ask their vendors if there is flexibility in the way data is presented on the screen.

💡 **Testing Tip**

Try searching for "sitagliptan," the generic name of Januvia. This drug was released in late 2006 and won't have any generic alternatives for a while.

❌ **Sometimes there is a slight lag in the interface between the server and the computer.** The mouse hangs on the screen, then suddenly moves. The button you clicked is activated and everything stops, only to start again a second or two later. It's as if the computer has petit mal seizures. You think you selected the right drug but the mouse click actually registered several entries higher or lower. In some cases, the selection window closes as soon as the click registers so you may not see what was actually selected for several screens.

Prevention: 🖊 **Users should double check their selections and take their time if the computer interface is slow or choppy.** They should upgrade their internet or server connection, or get a new computer if necessary.

 Pharmacist Perspective

⊕ **The pharmacist should always place the drug in the context of the patient's condition, patient instructions, dispense quantity, and refills.** Pharmacists should have a high sensitivity to anything that seems out of place and make a phone call to clarify. Errors in selection type will typically be very close to each other. The Confused Drug Names list published by the Institute for Safe Medication Practices is a good start.[117] In addition to look-alike spellings, a drug may be misselected simply due to proximity with another on an alphabetized list. Example: metoclopramide 10 mg tabs instead of metolazone 10 mg tabs.

(continues)

Pharmacist Perspective *(continued)*

Be sensitive to the drug category ordered. For example, Gurwitz and colleagues discovered in patients older than 65 years old that a few drug categories accounted for most of the preventable errors. From greatest to least frequency are: cardiovascular agents, diuretics, nonopioid analgesics, hypoglycemics, anticoagulants, and opioids.[118]

You Want Me to Put This Where?
The Fragile Nature of Formulations

The paper equivalent of choosing the wrong formulation on an e-prescription is best approximated when a route is confused. PO (by mouth) is misread as PR (rectally) or OU (both eyes). Many e-prescribing systems display all the commercially available formulations. Some formulations are appropriate for specialty practices or rare indications, though this is not evident from the selection screen. Powdered drug formulations, used only in compounding, appear between tablets, capsules, solutions, and injections. Consider the example of gentamicin 0.1% ointment and gentamicin 0.3% ointment. It can be difficult to distinguish the ophthalmic from the topical formulation. The 0.1% ointment is used topically. Unfortunately, the e-prescribing system may not give much more information than that.

Prevention: ⊕ **Users should work with their e-prescribing vendors to ensure the usual route for a formulation appears in the drug selection screen.** Better yet, they should ask for advanced filtering during drug selection as described in Chapter 4.

Testing Tip

Search for drugs with multiple indications used in multiple formulations such as hydrocortisone, ciprofloxacin and gentamicin. Can you clearly identify the drugs and their usual routes? Are they grouped together logically or are different formulations all mixed together?

I Should've Taken a Left at Albuquerque.
Choosing the Wrong Pharmacy

Selecting the wrong pharmacy is a new opportunity for error brought about by e-prescribing technology. Its closest paper cousin only surfaces when prescriptions are mailed or faxed to the wrong

---

🅡 **Pharmacist Perspective**

❗ **Wrong formulation is another big opportunity for error to creep in.**
On paper prescriptions, the prescriber writes the name of the drug, dose, and
route. This gives the pharmacist a great deal of freedom in choosing the best
formulation for the patient. Now, e-prescribing systems force the prescriber
to choose the formulation. The pharmacist should not assume the prescriber
knows what formulation is best. If the pharmacist has even a hint of a question, she should make the call. The initials that appear after drug names are
just as confusing for prescribers as they are to pharmacists. Was the order for
carbamazepine TC for therapeutic concentrate or tablet, chewable? That's a
big difference, especially since carbamazepine is available as a suspension
and not a therapeutic concentrate. The pharmacist should ask the prescriber
to clarify.

---

pharmacy; rarely do patients take their prescriptions to the wrong pharmacy.
Like medication lists in the e-prescribing system, it is easy to click on the
wrong pharmacy when the application displays a list of near-identical choices.
What are the consequences of choosing the wrong pharmacy? Patients may
have their therapy delayed and will certainly be frustrated if not upset. A large
proportion of medications can sustain a modest delay in therapy without ill
effect, especially medications being renewed (the patient presumably has a
supply). That still leaves a significant number of medications whose delay in
therapy can harm the patient; antibiotics, insulin, nitroglycerin, and beta
blockers represent a few examples.

Wrong Pharmacy

▽ **Prescriptions can end up in the wrong pharmacy when the
e-prescribing application remembers the last pharmacy at which the
prescription was filled.** Saving a patient's preference for pharmacy is a
great convenience until the patient wants the prescriptions sent to another
pharmacy. Consider the following hypothetical case constructed from actual
experiences:

> JH comes in on Friday afternoon to pick up her insulin prescriptions
> and the local pharmacy is the default pharmacy on her profile. JH had
> received insulin in the past through a mail-order pharmacy, but she
> now prefers the local pharmacy due to frustrations with the mail-order

(continues)

Wrong Pharmacy *(continued)*

pharmacy's shipping policies. JH asks for a new insulin prescription. The doctor renews the previous insulin orders and expects the prescription to go to the default pharmacy (the local pharmacy). Instead, the insulin goes to the mail-order pharmacy because that is where the prescription was sent last, regardless of the patient's current pharmacy preference. (The default pharmacy is only applied to new orders, not renewals.) JH is unable to get her insulin for several days and finally resorts to the emergency department for treatment.

As this case illustrates, the particular pharmacy applied to an order may depend on factors such as whether the order is new, whether it was sent to a pharmacy previously, and when the pharmacy preference was changed.

Prevention: **Solutions to prevent errors in pharmacy selection tend to be application specific.** Prescribers must take time to learn how their system handles pharmacies, including how they are added to the patient's profile, how they are remembered, and where the pharmacy is displayed in the profile. Prescribers should inform patients of usual expectations and instruct them (or the pharmacy) to call back for a reissue of prescriptions if the transmission is inadvertently diverted. Prescribers should place wording on their fax sheets to the pharmacy, if indicated, to call the office to verify prescriptions for patients not currently in the pharmacy's system. As an additional precaution, prescribers should place the name of the intended pharmacy on their fax sheets.

Testing Tip

Is the preferred pharmacy applied only to new orders, or is it applied to renewals as well? Does the pharmacy have to be selected every time, or is the information remembered as part of the order? Is the preferred pharmacy easily identified in the patient profile? Are local pharmacies and mail-order pharmacies present in your e-prescribing system? Can a pharmacy be added if it is not present in the displayed list?

Men Don't Take Birth Control Pills, Do They? Prescribing in the Wrong Patient's Profile

Prescribers sometimes talk about one patient's lab results while holding another patient's chart in their hands. Similarly, sometimes they write a

---

Pharmacist Perceptive

Pharmacists should always treat new prescriptions from unknown doctors for unknown patients with a healthy dose of skepticism. The chances are very good that they'll need more demographic information to complete the patient profile in the pharmacy computer. The pharmacist should take the opportunity to proactively call the medical office for the information instead of waiting for the patient to come in. He might uncover an error.

---

prescription for a husband while talking to his wife. Distractions can easily pull attention away for a moment and e-prescribing is just as vulnerable.

The e-prescribing application's interface and layout is important to preventing prescribing for the wrong patient. Users should note whether they can identify the patient's name at a glance, or if it is in a light-colored font tucked away in a corner and whether the patient's name is present on all the screens in the application. They should also notice whether the application allows multiple profiles to be open at the same time. These attributes and others contribute to the potential for error when prescribing.

Distractions aren't the only cause of prescribing in the wrong profile. The prescriber can select the wrong patient the same way he can select a wrong drug. Patient names should be displayed with other identifiers such as date of birth, address, and phone number. They should not be scrunched together in a small font on the screen.

Prevention: **Prescribers should develop a routine for resuming work after an interruption that includes verifying the patient's profile.** The routine should include completion of a five-point check anytime the prescriber's attention is drawn away in the middle of writing prescriptions.

Five-Point Check

To minimize the potential for error when resuming an interrupted task, the prescriber should ask himself these five questions:

1. What patient is active in the application?

2. For what patient am I intending to prescribe?

(continues)

Five-Point Check *(continued)*

3. Have I started writing a prescription?

4. What have I prescribed already?

5. What do I still need to prescribe?

Prescribers should force themselves to go through these questions after every interruption; their patients will be safer for it.

Pharmacist Perspective

❶ **A common situation for wrong patient selection is the husband/wife pairing or parent/child pairing.** It's obvious that the husband has no need of vaginal troches but matters are less clear when both husband and wife are on similar drugs. As with paper prescriptions, pharmacists must maintain a high sensitivity to medication orders that seem out of place with the rest of the patient's profile.

Clinical Case: A husband and wife were on an expensive brand-name blood pressure drug and requested prescriptions for an affordable generic equivalent. The husband took a dose twice as high as his wife's, and his blood pressure still wasn't controlled. The physician decided to increase his dose but erroneously converted the wife's prescription with the husband's dose in mind. The result was a fourfold increase in dose for the wife (but still within normal dose limits).

And . . . Poof! It's Gone! Cancelling out of an Order without Saving It

There it is, peeking out from the corner of a stack of charts—the prescription the prescriber swore had been put in the mail 3 days ago. The electronic equivalent is the order that is closed without saving. In many prescribing systems, there is a confirmation step before a prescription goes to the profile, printer, or pharmacy. It can be easy, especially after an interruption, to move on and inadvertently cancel work already done in a patient's profile.

Prevention: **The five-point checklist doubles as a useful tool for catching the premature cancellation error as well.** Many applications can generate a report of prescriptions written by a prescriber for the day. For prescribers who review this log regularly for accuracy, this error may come to light. Good practices aside, prescribers should take a moment to become familiar with the finishing options available. For those with paper charts, can a duplicate or nonlegal copy of the prescription be printed for the chart when they send or print the prescription? Does the application provide them with a message that indicates the prescription was sent or printed? Does the application resume an interrupted prescribing session or go back to its start page?

The Disappearing Act

Sometimes a prescription isn't received by the pharmacy even though the e-prescribing application indicates it was sent. This might be an indication of a connection issue with the pharmacy or a significant delay.

Delays in transmission can occur during the multiple exchanges required to successfully deliver the electronic prescription. Observe the lag time when sending prescriptions and note whether it is more prominent with prescriptions delivered as a fax than as an EDI transaction. If pharmacies that receive prescriptions as a fax consistently experience a delay, the solution may be to open dialogue with the pharmacy to encourage their adoption of an EDI capable solution. The infrastructure providers can be a resource for you on this matter.

Workflow and Process Challenges

The Patient Felt Fine Until He Woke Up Dead. Manual Entry Errors

A time comes when a patient or prescription or situation doesn't fit within the predefined categories of an e-prescribing application. It might be a lengthy patient instruction, an unusual drug, or a specific communication to the pharmacist. Whatever the case, it invariably requires manual entry—no mouse clicks, just straight typing. As with bad handwriting and poor spelling endemic with paper prescriptions, the potential for error rises dramatically when the prescriber takes words into her own hands. Lewis Carroll's line from *Alice in Wonderland,* "All mimsy were the borogroves, and the mome raths outgrabe," is perfectly readable and totally mystifying. The consolation prize of legibility offers no advantage to the unintelligible prescription.

A surprising number of e-prescribing applications do not allow entry of unrecognized drugs. On the surface, this sounds like a good idea, but it becomes problematic when trying to generate a prescription for home oxygen therapy, medical supplies, compounded medications, and investigational drugs. See also Chapter 4.

Patient instructions can be inflexible. Most e-prescribing applications will allow a user to type in specific patient directions, though exceptions abound here as well. Some applications force their structure on the patient instructions in addition to the free-text ability. The result is a confusing hybrid that promotes error. Instructions for warfarin 2 mg that should say "Take one tablet by mouth on even days alternating with one half tablet by mouth on odd days" might say "Warfarin 2 mg. Take one tablet daily as directed. Take one tablet by mouth on even days alternating with one half tablet by mouth on odd days."

This would indicate the application failed to suppress the rigid structure of patient instructions and failed to allow precedence to the more detailed free-text entry. Mashing both instructions together is a recipe for disaster.

Warning

A paper prescription is warranted if the e-prescribing application lacks the flexibility to safely represent complex patient instructions. Users should work with their vendors to resolve the issue. If it cannot be resolved in the near future (i.e., within the year), an alternate e-prescribing application should be considered.

If a prescriber does write the prescription on paper, he should be sure to enter the drug in the e-prescribing application in a generic manner so interaction checking will still occur. The prescriber should include a warning in the patient instructions such as "Do not dispense," to prevent it from being dispensed, should it accidentally be printed or sent to a pharmacy.

Prevention: **Prescribers should give their e-prescribing system a thorough workout with test prescriptions.** They must know how their prescriptions will appear on a fax machine and should work with a pharmacy to test a few e-prescribing transmissions. This identifies how their information appears at the pharmacy. They should check whether additional patient instructions are sent through the physician comments field, as well as where pharmacy comments appear on electronic renewal requests. Chapter 11 suggests that prescribers notify pharmacies that they have the ability to e-prescribe. This is exactly the kind of information pharmacies need to safely and efficiently process prescriptions. Notification materials are available at www.surescripts.com.

Testing Tip

Enter test prescriptions that have complex dosing and/or instructions such as warfarin, hydrocortisone cream, enoxaparin, or alendronate. Look at the prescription output. Is this what a pharmacist would see on a fax machine? Are the instructions clear? Does the application support half-tablet dosing? How does it handle the dose units for ointments, creams, eye drops, solutions, and injectables?

Pharmacist Perspective

℞ **Of all the information transmitted in an electronic prescription transaction, the patient instructions are the least mature.** Chapter 4 has more detail, but the technological limitations of patient instructions are important to note in this context. Pharmacy software applications have a system for rapidly entering patient instructions that developed independently of the e-prescribing applications that physicians use. The current NCPDP-SCRIPT standard sends patient instructions as a string of text that requires the pharmacist to reenter the information. Pharmacists should always check the physician comments field when processing e-prescriptions for medications that have complex dosing and/or instructions. The exact location of expanded patient instructions depends on the e-prescribing application. If expanded instructions aren't included in the usual field for transmission, the physician comments area is the next most widely used place.

The Medication That Wasn't. The Desire for Discontinuation Orders

Keeping a current active medication list is a problem with paper prescriptions and continues to be a problem with electronic prescriptions. Prompt documentation of discontinued medications is essential. This sleeper error becomes obvious during a patient admission to the hospital. All too often, the current medication list is printed from the electronic prescribing application. Without prompt documentation of discontinued orders, the patient is at risk for having inappropriate medications restarted on admission to the hospital.

To be fair, e-prescriptions have made great progress in making this good practice easier to do. Medications can be discontinued with a single click and many applications allow expirations to be placed on prescriptions, which will automatically discontinue them within the application.

Prevention: ⚕️ **Prescribers should use the discontinuation features present in their e-prescribing system.** Auto-discontinuation functions work well for short-term therapies such as antibiotics, pain relief, or conducting a trial on a new medication to evaluate a patient's tolerance for the therapy.

 Prescribers are advised to work with their vendor to allow annotations or comments (if that feature isn't already present) that document the reason a medication was discontinued, such as a patient's adverse reaction or because the medication was too expensive. This documentation is invaluable when making future therapeutic decisions and provides an incentive to discontinue medications correctly.

E-Rx users should work with their vendors to incorporate active alerts or reports that indicate when a medication is due for renewal. Lapse of a prescription may indicate the patient self-discontinued. Adherence alerts may help users stay informed about a patient's adherence and identify patients who may need to come in for evaluation.[71]

Prescribers should use the prescriber comments field in e-prescribing to tell the pharmacist if a previous medication has been replaced and why. For example, on an order for irbesartan, she might add, "Lisinopril is discontinued for cough," in the prescriber comments. This tells the pharmacist that the intention is to replace one medication with another. In addition, the pharmacist may note the reaction to lisinopril in the pharmacy system. There are conditions where coadministration of irbesartan and lisinopril is appropriate. By using the physician comments field, the prescriber avoids a phone call from the pharmacy for clarification at least, and she possibly prevents an error.

The ability to notify a pharmacy of a medication's cancellation or discontinuation is present in the NCPDP standard (CANRX) and is already used in some parts of the country. Optional certification for this transaction type is available for e-prescribing and pharmacy applications through SureScripts.

Some e-prescribing systems allow prescribers to create a free-text prescription in which they enter the name of a drug or supply "not recognized" in the application's database. Prescribers should take advantage of this function to create a message prescription and save it as a favorite. They can choose this message prescription and send it to the pharmacy as an interim measure until CANRX becomes available. See also Chapter 4. Such a sample prescription could look like this:

> **Drug Name: Message**
>
> **Patient Instructions: Discontinue [enter drug name here]**

Note: Those who use this strategy should avoid listing the name of the drug first, such as "Cipro D/C order." In the patient medication list, it could be mistaken for a drug order instead of a discontinuation order.

Meet My Frend, My Frind, My Freend, My Friend. Prescription Cloning 1, 2, 3

E-prescribing applications make it easy—almost too easy—to send prescriptions to a pharmacy. If a prescriber changes his mind about a prescription, the pharmacy could end up with multiple copies. Sorting out which prescription is most current challenges pharmacists and pharmacy staff and increases the potential for error. Pharmacy personnel will be left wondering which dose and drug are correct, and whether the prescriber intended to send two separate prescriptions or whether one replaces the other.

Cloning Confusion

A fax is received in a pharmacy and set aside. The prescription is changed by the prescriber and re-sent, but a different person in the pharmacy picks up the prescription. Someone sees the previous prescription and hands it to the pharmacist. Which came first? If the pharmacist is rushed, she may not notice the difference between time stamps on the fax (if there are any).

Prescribers' electronic prescriptions, if sent to a pharmacy fax, should contain fax header information. If they don't, the faxes mentioned in the sidebar are impossible to tell apart. The pharmacist is forced to call for clarification or risk making an error.

The same prevention strategies described in the section on proper discontinuation of orders apply to preventing errors due to cloned prescriptions.

Why Would Anyone Prescribe Vaginal Troches to be Taken by Mouth? The Indication for Indications

The practice of including indications on prescriptions is gaining momentum among prescribers, but is less consistent than it could be. The diagnosis or

---

Pharmacist Perspective

Pharmacists should check faxes for date/time stamps. If the date/time stamp is missing, it could be from an e-prescribing system. They should have a high sensitivity for multiple prescriptions of the same or similar drug received in a relatively short time frame. The potential for error is great and worth a call to the prescriber to clarify.

---

indication could easily be added to prescriptions but many applications have not developed tools for this. Most e-prescribing applications allow the entry of a problem or diagnosis in the patient's profile. Others go so far as to link the drug to the problem or diagnosis within the application. In a tragic lack of foresight, the crucial piece of information—the reason for which the drug is prescribed—often fails to reach the pharmacy.

 A prescription isn't dressed properly until it wears an indication. Without an indication, the pharmacy has no way of knowing if a beta-blocker prescription is for congestive heart failure, essential tremor, rate control, blood pressure, or migraine prophylaxis. Counseling patients on their prescriptions, a practice mandated by law in many states, becomes extremely difficult in the absence of an indication. Inappropriate counseling causes embarrassment to the pharmacist and possibly harm to the patient.

Prevention: ⊕ **The prescriber should always include the indication in the patient instructions of the prescription.** As discussed in Chapter 4, the ability of most applications to maintain a favorites list is quite useful. Prescribers can include indications in their list of commonly prescribed drugs and save themselves the task of retyping when they prescribe the same drug again. The question is whether to put the indication in the patient instruction field or the prescriber comments field. That depends on the e-prescribing application and how the favorites are saved. The application might link the diagnosis to the medication and relay that information to the pharmacy.

Designer Details

As an interim solution, application designers should consider copying a prescription's attached problem into the prescriber's comments field when the prescription is sent.

Prescribers can work with their vendor if their application doesn't currently allow that functionality.

Technology Challenges

The Computer Ate My Prescription. Detecting a Failed Transmission

Paper prescriptions are lost. The dog snacks on them; a child makes snowflakes with them; e-prescriptions disappear in an event called "failed transmission."

At least when a prescriber faxes a prescription, the fax machine tells him if the transmission was successful.

 E-prescribing applications address the issue of a failed transmission in a variety of ways, though few generate active alerts on a failed transmission. This passive approach increases potential for error and requires the prescriber (or nurse, secretary, office manager, or medical assistant) to monitor a report of failed transmissions. If needed, the failed transmissions can be re-sent. The causes of failed transmissions are many and usually temporary. Regardless, the end result is the same: a delay of therapy and a source of frustration.

Prevention: **It is important for prescribers to understand how their e-prescribing system handles failed transmissions and errors.** They should work with their vendor to implement an active alert system. In the meantime, they can put a process in place to check for failed transmissions regularly.

Pharmacist Perspective

Some of the causes of failed transmissions are due to the pharmacy applications. Good, common-sense practices are important; the pharmacy should keep paper in the fax machine, keep the phone lines open, and ensure the e-prescribing component of the pharmacy application is active and working. If the pharmacy staff does find a particular office routinely sends a deluge of prescriptions at the same time each day, they could be resolving their e-renewal requests at one time each day. Someone at the pharmacy could explain the effect it has on the pharmacy and offer to work on alternatives that work best for both parties. Everybody wins—the pharmacy, the prescriber, and especially the patients.

Click the Start Button to Stop.
When Standards Become Flexible

Strange and inconsistent behavior by an e-prescribing application breeds errors. The way standards are implemented within the application carries as much or more importance than the standards themselves. If the prescriber never sees the alert, errors happen. If renewing a medication takes 14 steps, errors happen. If the Send button tasks the nurse and the Print button sends the prescription to the pharmacy, errors happen.

Prevention: **Someone should test the e-prescribing application thoroughly before using it on a daily basis.** If that's not possible, users should document the idiosyncrasies as they are discovered and post the document where all the staff can see it. Communication is the best defense against errors from inconsistent application conventions. Users should review the document at staff meetings regularly—weekly during the first three months of implementation, then monthly for the next year. Someone in the office should work with the e-prescribing vendor to resolve the most troublesome issues.

Great Expectations, Hollow Results. The Dangers of Assumptions

Prescribers hand prescriptions to their patients with the expectation that the prescription will be taken to the pharmacy to be filled. Most do get filled, but a large number languish on nightstands, desks, or find their way to the trash. E-prescriptions eliminate the question of whether the prescription made it to the pharmacy, yet the expectation that it is filled is not always realized.

Every expectation is grounded in an assumption. The prescriber assumes all the information is sent correctly, but that assumption depends on the prescriber's knowledge of the e-prescribing application, standards, and normal conventions. Any number of errors can occur as a result of incomplete or inaccurate knowledge. There might not be an indication included on the prescription. Special instructions could be included in the prescriber comments, the patient instruction field, or some other place. The prescription might have gone to the pharmacy, or it might have gone to the nurse who is on vacation.

Prevention: **Understanding the transmission standards, best practices, and common e-prescribing conventions tempers assumptions and drives safety into one's prescribing habits.** Prescribers should monitor the prescription queue regularly to screen for dropped prescriptions and print a daily log of prescriptions generated. A quick, regular review of both reports should capture errors due to faulty assumptions.

Security Challenges

Free Prescriptions! Get 'Em While They're Hot!
Leaving the Application Unattended

Leaving an application unattended is akin to leaving a prescription pad on the table in the waiting room. People will avail themselves of the opportunity. Poor security opens the door for inadvertent (or intentional) prescribing done by someone else in the prescriber's name.

Prevention: **Prescribers should configure the system to prompt for a password to confirm prescriptions.** They should always log out when walking away from the system. Timed auto log-out options should be set, if that feature is available. The prescriber should review the daily report of prescriptions and be sure the prescriptions written are reasonable and familiar.

Technology Dependence

Drugs Have Relationships, Too.
The Truth about Interaction Checking

A clear advantage e-prescribing has over paper prescriptions is the ability to screen for drug interactions. These alerts tend to have the lowest override rates by prescribers.[64] This is a mixed blessing. Depending on the configuration, an e-prescribing application may not alert prescribers to significant interactions while other interactions, not so significant, are flagged. Nor is there great flexibility to adjust these configurations in many applications. The ability to screen drug interactions can be falsely reassuring.[64] The technology for clinical decision support is still evolving, as discussed in Chapter 7, but it can still be made to work to prescribers' benefit.

Prevention: **⊕ There's no substitute for clinical knowledge.** Prescribers must know the major drug interactions. They can use the drug interaction alert flags as a guide and reminder, not a substitute. Many applications allow prescribers to adjust clinical alert settings. This allows prescribers to find the best configuration that balances the number of significant alerts against the presence of alerts that are not meaningful.

If the application has the flexibility to customize alerts, prescribers should work with a pharmacist to define alerts requiring intervention. The combined effort may be more successful than working alone and serve to reduce alert fatigue while increasing patient safety.[47]

Clinical Communications

As Grizzle and colleagues showed,[119] documentation of a reason for a drug–drug interaction override is helpful, if the application allows. Pharmacists find the following reasons particularly useful:

- The basis for the route of medication administration.

- Presence of active monitoring to prevent or ameliorate the consequences of a given drug–drug interaction.

- The action the prescriber will take in consideration of the interaction.

- Information to the effect that the patient was not taking one of the interacting drugs.

- Any other clear communication that adequately addresses the clinical concern.

 Testing Tip

Enter test prescriptions for warfarin, simvastatin, diltiazem, aspirin, and sulfamethoxazole/trimethoprim to evaluate how robust the alerts are. See Appendix C for the full panel of orders to enter to give the application a good workout.

Computers Are Good at Math, Right? Auto-Calculate Quandaries

Quantity and day's supply are manually calculated and written on paper prescriptions. E-prescribing applications provide some convenience by doing those calculations for the users. Again, this is a mixed blessing. Some medications, especially the liquids, injectables, and topicals, are prone to misapplied logic in software systems. For example, one may find that an order for prefilled enoxaparin 40 mg syringes will automatically calculate very differently depending on whether milligrams, milliliters, or dose units are used.

The true test of the application is its answer to this simple question: Can the user enter the correct amount? Some applications insist on replacing the correct value with their incorrect value. Other applications don't have the correct units to express what is needed. In the preceding example, it would be nice to dispense 10 prefilled enoxaparin syringes. Does the application allow the prescriber to prescribe 10 syringes, or is she stuck with a generic term like units that could cause errors?

E-prescribing applications will apply the auto-calculate logic in what appears to be an inconsistent manner. (There is a logic that explains the behavior, it's just not expected by the prescriber.) Does the auto-calculate function activate when an existing order is altered? What if, for example, the frequency changes from twice daily to three times daily? Does the application automatically calculate in both directions? That is, if the prescriber changes the day's supply, does the dispense quantity change? Does the user get auto-calculate functionality multiple times on the same prescription? In other words, if the prescriber can't make up his mind and changes the frequency three times, does the dispense quantity change three times?

Some medications are dispensed as whole units even though partial doses are used. Prefilled syringes, such as those with insulin and heparin, are the most common example. Can the application handle orders where a partial dose is prescribed but whole units need to be dispensed?

Testing Tip

The tester should enter sample prescriptions that have unusual dosing units such as hydrocortisone cream, enoxaparin, albuterol solution for nebulizer, phenytoin suspension, and lindane shampoo. Appendix C also lists test prescriptions.

Pharmacist Perspective

Quantity is another area in which a pharmacist should develop a high sensitivity and low tolerance for strangeness. Auto-calculation functions are still maturing, and the chances that something may be incorrect with the quantity are high. Anything that doesn't appear to match well with the patient directions should be clarified with the prescriber. For example: an order indicates dispense No. 60 for a medication taken three times daily. Was the patient taking it twice daily before? Does the prescriber really want a 20-day supply?

Sometimes the auto-calculate function is disabled when the user manually enters a number. In that case, the user should be sure the numbers don't become transposed to avoid entering a prescription error such as a dispense quantity of one with 30 refills.

Prevention: ⚕**Prescribers should make a point of understanding how auto-calculate functions activate in their e-prescribing application.** They should always double check the final prescription to see if it looks reasonable and adjust dose alerts, if needed. The dose alerts will often catch entry errors in day's supply and quantity.

Make Up My Mind Already. Finessing Fickle Formularies

Patients who pay less for their prescriptions tend to be more adherent with their therapy. Sometimes the best drug isn't the best drug, it's the one the patient will take. Formulary suggestions can help find that drug.

❶ Like many features and technologies, formularies are maturing as well, though providing useful alternatives is where the largest share of work is needed. For example, when writing for sustained-release oxycodone, the prescriber may find methadone listed at the top of a suggested alternative list. See also Chapter 4.

❶ Another interesting quirk of formularies is uncovered through the Dispense As Written, or DAW, box. A branded medication can be selected and flagged as a preferred medication for that insurance plan since a generic is available. On selecting DAW, one would expect the formulary status to change to a nonpreferred or uncovered brand. In many e-prescribing applications, the preferred status stays even though the prescription for the brand is a substantially higher cost to the insurer and the patient.

 Testing Tip

Enter a prescription for Plendil and note the formulary status. Most plans should give this a green light as the generic felodipine is widely available. Now enter the prescription over again and this time mark the DAW box. Did the formulary status change?

Prevention: ⚕ **Prescribers can't assume the agents listed are clinical suggestions or valid therapeutic alternatives.** They must make their choice based on what is best for the patient.

Pharmacist Perspective

Giving the prescribers access to the formulary is one of the best advances e-prescribing has put forth. The effect it has on e-prescriptions can be seen in the choice of drug. Some prescribers choose drugs from the suggested alternates list that are not appropriate or choose rare formulations that are not readily available. When received as an e-prescription, the odds are good this is more an issue with the e-prescribing application than the prescriber. A call to the prescriber along with a little education can go a long way for making future prescriptions go smoother for both the prescriber and the pharmacist.

Clinical Challenges

The Blue Pill or the Red Pill? Why Isn't There a Yellow? Prescribing an Overdose or Underdose

Paper systems offer no protection against errors in prescribing overdoses or underdoses. While e-prescribing systems are making headway, many lack the sophistication to warn of a true underdose or overdose; more than half of prescribing errors are dosing errors.[75] The maturation of clinical decision support and higher-level integration of e-prescribing into larger health information networks will allow a better solution than is generally available at the present time. Most current applications cannot place the dose into a clinical context that accounts for age, concomitant diseases, indication, or organ function. See also Chapters 6 and 7.

Prevention: **Prescribers should test their system to see how underdoses and overdoses with medications such as acetaminophen, warfarin, and amoxicillin are handled.** They should investigate where and how upper and lower dose limits are applied in the system. Does the e-prescribing application allow prescribers to set their own limits in addition to the standard configuration?

Pharmacist Perspective

Dose checking is a feature that is currently drug specific, not patient specific. Clinicians will still need to perform manual dose checking on e-prescriptions to ensure the medication is appropriate for the patient.

Prescribers should work with their e-prescribing vendor to turn off alerts that offer no information, such as an alert flag that reads, "Dosing information is not available." Such messages only contribute to alert fatigue and increase the chance that an important alert will be ignored.

His Kidneys Needed the Exercise.
Adjusting the Dose for Kidney Function

Most e-prescribing systems are not integrated with lab values and lack the ability to inform a prescriber of a medication that needs to be adjusted for renal function. The maturation of clinical decision support and higher-level integration of e-prescribing into larger health information networks will allow a better solution than is generally available at the present time.

Prevention: A prescriber must know a patient's renal function when prescribing and adjust appropriately.

Conclusion

E-prescribing is safer than paper prescriptions, and yet, as this chapter demonstrates, the opportunity for error is still alive and well despite the improvement in safety. Errors occur in ways that are highly improbable. As such, our ability to prevent error is limited only by our inability to anticipate error. Implementing the prevention strategies outlined in this chapter will help prevent potential errors from becoming real errors.

PART IV

Implementation

How to Assess for E-Prescribing Readiness

This chapter and the next two chapters address the challenges of implementing e-prescribing in the outpatient setting. The transition to e-prescribing passes through four stages: assessment, planning, implementation, and evaluation. Assessment asks the preliminary questions. What resources are needed in the office to support e-prescribing? Who will drive the process? How will the workflow need to change? One way or another, these questions are resolved with every transition to e-prescribing. Answering them before the first prescription flies through cyberspace makes the transition to e-prescribing smoother, promotes safety for patients, and enhances staff satisfaction.

Chapters 11 and 12 address planning, implementation, and evaluation. Planning takes the information from assessment and imposes an order. Investing time in planning pays dividends in a speedy implementation plagued with few problems. Implementation puts the plan into action while evaluation checks to make sure the plan is the right one.

> **(Rx) Pharmacist Perspective**
>
> Implementation of e-prescribing in a pharmacy may be easier than imple-
> menting such a system in a doctor's office. Pharmacy applications have been
> electronic for years and the established workflows change little with
> e-prescriptions. In most cases, implementing e-prescribing in the pharmacy
> is similar to a software upgrade to the dispensing application. Contrast this
> with a fundamental shift from paper systems to electronic applications that
> prescribers experience when adopting e-prescribing.

The Triad

In an ideal world, e-prescribing is implemented in an environmental triad of the
right resources, skills, and culture. All three elements are needed in sufficient
quantities for the transition to e-prescribing to be successful.[72] If an office has the
personnel skills and a culture ready for e-prescribing but has no equipment, time,
or staff to support it, implementation fails.[95] If an office has motivated employees with the right equipment but no one knows how to use the technology or
manage change, implementation fails. If an office has the right people and equipment but no one wants to change or use the technology, implementation fails.

The assessment phase brings these challenges into the open where they can
be addressed.[120] A path to e-prescribing can be blazed over, around, or
through the obstacles revealed by the assessment. Resources in one area can
be leveraged to overcome deficiencies in another.

Right Resources

Having the right resources is the first element of the triad. The resources most
relevant to the systems affecting e-prescribing are time, staff, equipment, and
expert knowledge. Deficiencies in any of these extend the time it takes to successfully complete a transition to e-prescribing. If the deficiency is severe
enough, the transition may never be complete.

Time—The Challenge

Time is a commodity always in short supply. Though e-prescribing may save
time, the transition consumes time in the form of training and practice. The
amount of time consumed depends on the e-prescribing application, staff

familiarity with the technology, training options available, and other variables. Managers should plan on 4 hours of training and 4 hours of practice for each staff member. Any time not used can be repurposed for troubleshooting or extended training for other staff.

Answering the following questions can help managers assess their time resources:

- Do you have enough time in your daily schedule to accommodate training?
- Do you have enough time for retraining?
- Do you have time to absorb slowdowns from workflow changes?
- Do you have staff time to enter patient demographics or past medication orders?[18]

Challenges to the time resource are not always due to a deficiency of supply; sometimes the availability of time is variable or unstable. A call from the hospital or the arrival of a sick patient disrupts the best laid plans. Personnel in the office may have an available hour that is broken into 10- and 15-minute chunks scattered through the day.

Time—What to Do

Time can be managed in a number of creative ways that should be individualized for the office. Some suggestions include:

After Hours: Extend the workday. Temporarily staggering the arrival of staff in the morning allows late-arriving staff to stay later without incurring overtime. Are all staff needed at 8 a.m. or can one person come in at 9 a.m. and work an hour later? The extra daily hour squeezed out by this rotation can be used for both training and data entry.

The negative consequences of this strategy should also be considered. Some staff, such as those who open and close the office, may work longer during the entire transition. Not all staff have flexibility in their home life to accommodate a change in their work schedules. Babysitters and bus routes disrupt carefully planned schedules in unpredictable ways. If offsetting shifts isn't feasible, overtime or additional time is an option.

Scheduling: Managers should plan for a 25% reduction in patient volume for the 2 weeks surrounding implementation. Staff should schedule one fewer patient per hour than usual to allow time for training and adjusting to different workflows. Knowing the time is available may help to lower stress levels and ease the transition. For staff, the reduction in workload speaks of a commitment to the e-prescribing technology, makes the task achievable, and psychologically prepares them for success.

Another strategy is to schedule patients in a way that creates room in the day. Perhaps complete physicals can be done on one day in the week. Maybe visit slots for acute and urgent patients can be moved to the end of the day. Managers should consider the types of patients that consume the most time and those who are the most unpredictable. They should try to find a way to organize those patients in the schedule to allow breathing room for the transition to e-prescribing.

Training: Dividing the training into smaller segments makes it easier to fit into the spaces of the workday. Training should be flexible. Different training methods might be particularly suited to a particular office. Computer-based training and self-learning may be sufficient for most of the staff while some may need one-on-one instruction. If more comprehensive instruction is needed, perhaps a single member in the office can be trained thoroughly, and that person can, in turn, train the others. This is called the train-the-trainer approach.

Supplemental Staff: Hiring supplemental staff to assist in the data entry tasks or to cover job functions for staff involved in training is another way to gain time.

Pharmacist Perspective

The time needed to train in the pharmacy is relatively small compared to the prescriber's environment. Scheduling the training becomes the largest challenge; per diem staff and float personnel cannot be overlooked. These staff frequently work weekends and off hours—times when the potential for error is high.

Staff—The Challenge

People are the resources that drive e-prescribing; prescribers write e-prescriptions, their staff process renewals, pharmacists fill prescriptions, and patients take the medications. The process grinds to a lurching halt if people are missing. A staff shortage is a huge barrier to a successful transition to e-prescribing. The shortage could be chronic, such as an unfilled position in the office, or acute, such as someone who calls in sick on the day of training. Regardless of the cause, the effect is the same: a busy day for the office. Training in this environment is less than optimal. The obligation to answer phones or attend to patients shreds any attempt at learning.

Staff: What to Do

As with the challenges to time, supplemental staff may be a short-term fix. If the problem is chronic in nature, a better solution may be to wait until the positions are filled. Implementing change in an office filled with overworked staff is like going to exercise at the gym after finishing a triathlon. Change requires full staff resources for a safe transition.

One suggestion is to investigate a staffing swap with an office that is already e-prescribing. Swapping a secretary or nurse on a temporary basis brings expertise into your office and provides your staff an opportunity to learn an electronic system. For larger health systems that have a float pool of personnel who already circulate through owned practices, this may represent an efficient way to support and educate personnel throughout the implementation.

The Unique Challenge

Sharing staff with another office is a great opportunity to bring best practices into your own office. Take a moment to explicitly state your expectations to staff traveling to a different office. Staff may believe their office is unique and fail to bring back practices and ideas that could be beneficial.

Equipment—The Challenge

E-prescribing is a new technology that requires equipment to function the way a pen requires ink to write. At a minimum, a computer, printer, and internet connection are needed. The computer in this sense represents any device that runs the e-prescribing application such as a PDA, tablet, personal computer, cell phone, or other device. The printer is needed to print prescriptions for controlled substances, prescriptions that require hard copy (some Medicaid regulations require this), and to honor patient requests for paper prescriptions. The most obvious challenge confronting implementation is the lack of equipment. Managers considering implementing an e-prescribing system should ask themselves the following questions:

- If the equipment is present, is it outdated?
- If the equipment is current, does it need maintenance or repair?

If the answer to either of those questions is yes, this indicates a resource challenge that can paralyze the transition. Depending on office requirements, additional equipment, such as a wireless network or fax server, may be needed.

Hale has an excellent section on the requirements necessary for e-prescribing, both for hardware and contracting needs.[38]

Equipment–What to Do

Once equipment needs are known, managers should create a budget that includes upgrades to the existing equipment, maintenance, and repair costs. Internet access is a revolving expense while the printer and computers are usually up-front costs. A wireless network is a convenience, but it may not be required depending on workflow. If expenses are tight, an investment in redesigning work-flows could save money on the hardware cost. Many internet service providers can assist with obtaining the right equipment and setting up a network.

Expert Knowledge–The Challenge

Ongoing use of e-prescribing requires a person proficient and familiar with the application who can serve as a special resource. Unlike previous resources, a total lack of expert knowledge won't derail the transition to e-prescribing, but its presence is helpful.

Expert Knowledge–What to Do

Consider creating a local expert role within the office and plan for the appropriate training. The expert could be the trainer in the train-the-trainer approach, or the office manager, or the prescriber. Regardless of the person chosen, training someone to this level of proficiency creates a valuable on-site resource.

Not every office has a person able to become the expert. In those situations, the availability of a robust support service is critical and should be explored before committing to a specific e-prescribing application.

Managers considering an e-prescribing system should find out whether the vendor provides technical support, and ask the following questions:

- How much does it cost?
- When is it available?
- What is the vendor's turnaround time on issues?

Pharmacist Perspective

Access to expert knowledge is just as important in the pharmacy as it is in the medical office or hospital. The expert can help find out why a renewal request didn't get processed and how a prescription for an odd formulation should be handled. The expert facilitates operations like oil between gears.

Right Skills

A critical deficiency in the necessary skills will cripple an implementation process even with all the right resources present. Three sets of skills are needed during the transition to e-prescribing: basic computer skills, workflow skills, and personnel skills. Of the three, basic computer skills carry the most weight.

Basic Computer Skills—The Challenge

E-prescribing requires a computer, and the need for basic skills extends beyond the prescriber. These skills include turning the computer on, using a mouse, opening and closing application windows, moving files around, copying and pasting text, and using an internet browser. Someone who has never used a computer will find e-prescribing doubly challenging—the conventions of the computer must be learned in addition to the conventions of the e-prescribing application.

People may lack basic computer skills for different reasons. A person may have had no need to use a computer prior to this point, may be uncomfortable with the technology, or may simply be unskilled.

Perplexing Patterns

People have remarkable adaptation skills that allow them to function in environments without a true understanding of the job they perform. The following case study shows an example. During an upgrade to a newer version of software in a pharmacy, the icons on the employees' desktops became rearranged. As a result, several of the staff were unable to function the morning of the upgrade. The application wasn't gone, but the staff didn't know how to find the program on the hard drive. They had memorized the patterns of actions needed for their jobs but failed to gain any deeper understanding that would've allowed effective troubleshooting.

Staff may be familiar with the hardware pieces of computers—the mouse, keyboard, monitor, and a few basic software functions—but lack an understanding of the common conventions at work within the computer. They may have no formal computer training or have received training as needed. Someone told them to click on an application icon, another person showed them how to close a window.

Before beginning training with these individuals, it's important to address their fears and concerns. Many are afraid of doing permanent damage to the computer or application. Once the emotional aspect of technology is engaged, actual learning can begin.

Other staff, though familiar and skilled with computers, may be uncomfortable. They remain reluctant to use the computer unless absolutely necessary. This creates a functional skill deficit, though they potentially may learn the e-prescribing application more quickly than individuals without any computer experience.

Basic Computer Skills—What to Do

Remedial training is appropriate for the person lacking basic computer skills. Local colleges, universities, and libraries offer classes at a reasonable cost and sometimes for free. If you are a part of a large health system, the internal education department may have training available. The sooner this need is identified, the better. The time used to develop familiarity with the computer before e-prescribing implementation will only help the process.[121]

The person who uses pattern recognition may also benefit from remedial training, though a few may have difficulty with the concepts involved. For these people, prolonging remedial training may be effective at teaching the necessary skills. Depending on the person's role, redesigning the office workflows may be easier than requiring the individual to function in a capacity for which she is prone to error.

Redesigning workflows is a strategy that can circumvent a person's lack of basic computer skills. If the nurse has difficulty printing patient education handouts, perhaps the task can be done by the medical assistant or at patient checkout. Altering workflows can take different forms in every office with varying degrees of efficiency. In one office, the prescriber wanted to preserve the existing workflow and insisted the staff transcribe the written prescriptions into the e-prescribing application. This kind of workflow introduces more systems into the process and increases the potential for error.

Redesigned Workflow

An office had a secretary who lacked basic computer skills and functioned solely on pattern recognition. The original workflow called for the office secretary to use the e-prescribing application when patients requested a prescription renewal. Patients tended to be vague when describing their medications,

(continues)

Redesigned Workflow *(continued)*

and having the list available to the secretary would help to determine which prescription needed renewing so the nurse or doctor could be made aware. The revised workflow had the secretary direct the patient to call the pharmacy for renewal requests. This eliminated the need for the secretary to interact with the e-prescribing application. In the end, using the pharmacy to generate a renewal request proved to be more efficient and, by eliminating a number of intermediate systems, decreased the potential error.

There is no right or wrong workflow. One prescriber restricted e-prescribing to himself, and other office staff were not involved in the prescribing workflow at all. This reduced the number of systems affecting prescriptions and allowed the prescriber to thoroughly learn the e-prescribing software. However, the choice to exclude other staff also limited workflow options that could have offered greater efficiencies (renewal processing) and safety (enhanced access to the patients' medication lists).

 Pharmacist Perspective

Pharmacies can assist the medical office in addressing workflow challenges as the convention of asking the patient to call the pharmacy for renewals demonstrates. The degree to which the pharmacy can help depends on the relationship with the medical office. The pharmacy might be an exclusive provider for a particular patient population, such as hospice or home infusion, or it might be one of many others with which the medical office deals. The closer the relationship, the more the pharmacy should be involved with the transition to e-prescribing.

Workflow Skills—The Challenge

Learning new workflows is responsible for the majority of change experienced in the office. An individual adept at problem solving and managing change keeps processes running smoothly. Conversely, an individual who has difficulty problem solving and managing change hinders the transition. This individual is unsure what to do when the password isn't accepted, when nothing prints, or when the pharmacy calls to say it didn't receive the prescription. Someone skilled with change management will check the Caps Lock key, ensure the printer has paper, or pull up the e-prescribing transmission log.

Workflow Skills—What to Do

Poor workflow skills in the office are a powerful incentive to automate workflows as much as possible. This approach shifts work away from a known weakness—poor change management. This may require investing in additional technology such as a fax server, wireless network, or new computers. Spending time planning and defining the workflows assists in overcoming this challenge as well. Involving staff in discussions of the proposed office workflows actively engages the entire office with the result that proposed solutions are more likely to be accepted.

 Pharmacist Perspective

E-prescribing workflow in the pharmacy is nearly transparent. Variations in implementation are worth exploring, however. Are renewals automatically sent electronically to prescribers or does the pharmacist need to choose the delivery option? Do new e-prescriptions appear in a queue for the pharmacist or do they interrupt the current prescription in progress? The answers to these questions determine the degree to which the pharmacist's workflow is affected. How adept are pharmacy staff at troubleshooting these functions?

Personnel Skills—The Challenge

Making the change to electronic prescribing requires a good understanding of staff abilities and staff perspectives; it also requires an understanding of the emotional impact the change is likely to have.[20] A person with good personnel skills applies this understanding throughout the implementation process. Unlike the skills previously discussed, good personnel skills don't need to be present in every person, though it would certainly be helpful.[122] A person insensitive to personnel issues will have a difficult time planning and implementing electronic prescribing; conflict within the office is inevitable.

Personnel Skills—What to Do

Several techniques can overcome the limitations imposed by a deficiency in good personnel skills. First and foremost, managers should enhance good communication; they should hold regular meetings with the staff to discuss the implementation process and use memos or other written communication to keep staff informed. If time is tight, clear out the lunch hour to have discussions about the transition. An e-prescribing champion within the office may provide the sensitivity and assistance necessary to engage the staff. The champion doesn't have to be an expert, just a person motivated and committed to seeing e-prescribing implementation continue successfully. The champion is the moral support for the transition and the point person for staff to go to with concerns. The champion facilitates all aspects of the implementation process.

 Pharmacist Perspective

Communication is always a good idea no matter the environment. Posting key process changes in relevant areas such as the fax machine and order entry stations go a long way to facilitating adherence with the new processes. Different prescribers using different applications will have small variations in the way prescriptions present. How are those variations communicated to the pharmacy staff? Posting a change log in a publicly accessible place is one way to ensure all staff are current with new processes, troubleshooting tips, and policy changes.

Right Culture

Having the right culture facilitates a successful transition to e-prescribing[13] and comprises the last element of the triad. The best resources and skills cannot overcome a culture resistant to change. The milder form of this resistance is nonaction or passive resistance. This is the unengaged person who goes through the motions during training (if he shows up), asks no questions, voices no concerns directly, and volunteers for nothing. During lunches or smoking breaks, this person might complain about the process and produce an amazing array of reasons for keeping things the same.

A rarer, more dangerous form of resistance is the person who takes an active role, intentionally sabotaging efforts towards e-prescribing. Communications are misplaced or dropped by this person; misunderstanding is the rule rather than the exception, and problems with equipment needed for e-prescribing go unreported. How do you handle these people? How can they be brought on board to participate in the implementation and change in workflow? Druskat and Wolff have an excellent article on team building and the emotional intelligence of groups that may help.[122]

Persuading Prescribers

Three prescriber attitudes may be encountered when initiating change, nicely summed up by Dr. LeTourneau as follows:

- I will be perceived as incompetent.
- This is going to interfere with getting my work done.
- I don't know what this is or why it's being proposed.

Consider addressing the prescriber's fear of the unknown and perceived incompetence with information, training, and a position of control throughout the implementation process.[123]

The culture challenge is summed up as facing unwillingness to change, inability to accept change, or inability to sustain change. The permanent solution may be ongoing in nature and beyond the scope of transitioning to e-prescribing. Short-term solutions may carry a recalcitrant individual through the change transition even though she may not be fully reconciled to the change.

Involving staff early in the process helps to address many of the fears a person may have. Actively soliciting feedback instead of waiting for people to step forward with ideas, questions, or concerns engages all members of the office. Specific emotional and educational needs can be dealt with more effectively before implementation begins.

Pharmacist Perspective

This awareness and attention to the human dynamic is also needed in the pharmacy. Encouraging a positive work culture is an ongoing activity with benefits beyond the implementation of e-prescribing.

Conclusion

This chapter crossed multiple disciplines and areas of study. The suggested approaches may be adequate for a large number of offices, but severe deficiencies in any area may still require specialized solutions. A consultant knowledgeable in the particular area of need should be engaged if an assessment reveals a serious deficiency. If hardware is needed, the office manager should consult with an information technology professional. If the office culture is intensely negative, a consultant who handles group and team dynamics may be needed.

Performing an assessment, formal or informal, provides guidance for planning and implementation. Mentally reviewing the issues described in the chapter and applying the situations to the people involved in e-prescribing may be sufficient for some offices. Other offices may prefer a more formal approach. Appendix E contain tools to assist with the assessment process.

Regardless of the manner in which the assessment is done, the results directly affect the implementation process. The implementation date may need to be postponed if the assessment reveals critical deficiencies that need attention. If external forces impose upon the implementation date, the assessment may raise awareness of potential issues during implementation. Knowing what might be a problem is needed to prevent the problem.

Chapter 11

How to Implement E-Prescribing

READING PRIORITY

Implementation puts the information from assessment to good use. This is where the rubber hits the road or, in the case of e-prescribing, where the prescription hits the computer.

This first part of this chapter covers the planning needs for training, disaster preparedness, and the ways in which communication, prescribing, and administrative functions may change. We'll discuss questions that need answering and the tasks involved in implementation. The second part of this chapter expands on the planning phase and marshals the planning energy into the 4 to 6 weeks prior to implementation, specifically addressing the ways the office can overcome the twin obstacles of demographic and historical data entry.

Planning

For organization and clarity, we'll discuss the planning stage as four large areas: staff roles, application configuration, training, and disaster preparedness. The office will confront questions in these areas and the answers require a good understanding of current processes. E-prescribing offers new ways of getting the same work done, eliminates other work, and enables the provision of new services that weren't feasible before. To take full advantage of the benefits e-prescribing offers, constantly challenge yourself to identify the reason why existing processes are the way they are. You can use the worksheets in the appendices to identify your existing workflows and develop a crosswalk to the new workflow under e-prescribing.

Example

Perhaps the existing workflow calls for a copy of the written prescription to be faxed to a nurse in a long-term care facility for nursing home patients. Is a copy of the prescription needed for the nurse if she has access to the e-prescribing application? Is an active medication list needed in both the chart and the e-prescribing application? Providing access to the e-prescribing application for appropriate users may eliminate entire paper-based workflows.

Those planning a conversion to e-prescribing should allow at least 4 weeks before the intended implementation to find answers for difficult questions and perform any preparatory work needed. The time isn't mandatory, but it is prudent. The extra time makes implementation as problem free as possible.[115]

Planners should give consideration to the overall structure and scalability of implementation. Different approaches to implementation include those that are:

- *Comprehensive*: The entire office is engaged and trained for e-prescribing.

- *Vertical*: A single doctor, nurse, and/or secretary within the office pilot the e-prescribing process. Workflows are refined within this functional unit before the rest of the office is engaged in e-prescribing.

- *Horizontal*: Only the prescribers pilot the e-prescribing process, assuming responsibility for all e-prescribing functions. As their comfort level grows with the application, the workflows expand to include nurses. In the last step, the workflows expand to include the secretaries.

Staff Roles

Communication

The prescription process involves communication in nearly every aspect from patient to secretary to nurse to physician to pharmacist. E-prescribing offers a radically different way to communicate through this process. As a result, several key workflows need to be thought through prior to implementation to ensure the continuance of smooth operations.

Renewal Requests
Patients and pharmacies communicate the need to renew prescriptions through a variety of channels including by telephone, by fax, through representatives, and in person. E-prescribing offers an additional means of communication. Consider how the current workflow for managing prescription renewal requests may change with the presence of e-prescribing by asking the following questions:

- How will faxed requests for renewals be handled? Attention to this workflow, as detailed in **Table 11.1**, is needed to avoid increasing the potential for error. See also the example in Appendix E.

- How will e-renewal requests be handled?

    ○ Will the prescriber view all e-renewals and forward them to a nurse or secretary for processing? Conversely, will the nurse or secretary process e-renewals and forward them to the prescriber for authorization?

    ○ Are different workflows needed for different e-renewal requests such as controlled substances versus noncontrolled substances or maintenance versus acute medications?

- How will phoned patient requests for prescription renewals be handled?

    ○ Will the secretary queue prescriptions for the prescriber to renew?

    ○ Will the patient be referred to the pharmacy?

    ○ Will the call be forwarded to the nurse for processing?

- How will patient requests for prescription renewals be handled when the patient presents for a visit?

    ○ Will the secretary or nurse preemptively ask if any prescriptions need renewing?

    ○ Will renewals be handled during the patient visit or after the visit?

Patient Education
E-prescribing provides the option to print patient information regarding the prescriptions written. This is especially useful when samples are dispensed since this action bypasses the counseling and written information pharmacies

TABLE 11.1 Responses to Faxed Prescription Renewal Requests

Action	Advantages	Disadvantages
Fax or phone a request to the pharmacy to provide an e-renewal	Future faxed requests may be prevented E-prescribing workflows are preserved May uncover an educational opportunity. For example, reasons why the pharmacy is unable to send e-renewal requests can be investigated. This may lead to adjustments in either application, resulting in future e-renewals; demonstrate the importance of the e-renewals to the pharmacy resulting in acquisition of e-renewal capability; or simply provide a better understanding of the process used by the pharmacy to request renewals.	This is an extra step that takes more time.
Renew the medication within the e-prescribing application	Expedient E-prescribing workflows are preserved	Does not prevent future faxed requests or increase e-renewals; trades short-term expediency at the expense of an efficient, lasting solution.
Fax or phone the renewal to the pharmacy	Expedient	Double work. The medication still needs to be entered in the prescriber's e-prescribing application to maintain an accurate medication list. Otherwise, the patient's medication profile becomes outdated and changes into a chimeric combination of paper and electronic records that increases the potential for error. Does not prevent future faxed requests or increase e-renewals; trades short-term expediency at the expense of an efficient, lasting solution.

Fast Fax Fixes

Until health care is further along the technological highway, faxed requests for prescription renewals from pharmacies, though reduced with e-prescribing, will still occur. What options are available to the office for managing these?

First, one must identify whether the prescription can be sent electronically or not. Controlled substances and prescriptions that require an inked signature cannot be sent electronically. Table 11.1 describes possible actions and their consequences for prescriptions that can be sent electronically.

---

provide. If patient education is to be generated in the office, one must address these workflow questions:

- Where are the computer and printer resources?

  - Are computers and printers available throughout the office or only in certain areas?

- Who will print patient education materials and when?

  - Will the nurse print the information at check-in?

  - Will the prescriber print information during the visit?

  - Will the secretary print information at patient checkout?

Pharmacy Perspective

Many pharmacy applications will send or give the option to send renewal requests electronically if an office is identified as capable of receiving electronic prescriptions. How does the pharmacy application know if the prescriber can receive electronic renewal requests? That information is kept updated by infrastructure providers such as SureScripts and others. Most pharmacy applications automatically update the list of local prescribers that can receive these e-renewals. If a pharmacist finds that prescribers can receive e-renewal requests but are not flagged in the pharmacy application as such, the pharmacist should contact her vendor. There are a number of rare circumstances that could result in this situation, and troubleshooting the matter with the vendor will be most efficient.

Medication Effectiveness

Some e-prescribing applications allow documentation of therapy effectiveness, which provides several benefits. Medical justification for the current therapy is easier, reasons for medication discontinuation enable better choices for future therapies, and communication with other healthcare providers is facilitated when making therapy changes. For example, a patient calls with a complaint of diarrhea from a sample medication given at the last visit. The prescriber discontinues the medication and documents a reason of GI intolerance.

Other communication features in e-prescribing applications, such as tasking and annotations, make scribbled sticky notes nearly obsolete. To take full advantage of these features, those planning an e-prescribing implementation should consider these workflow questions:

- What information will be internally communicated or documented by the e-prescribing application?

  ○ Patient's response to therapy, good or bad?

  ○ Special patient needs such as impending travel plans, unusual insurance coverage, or caregiver concerns?

  ○ Reason for medication discontinuation or change?

- How will these communication options change office workflows? For example:

  ○ Will the secretary forward a patient's phone call to the nurse, or will a task for the nurse be generated?

  ○ Will the nurse interrupt the prescriber during a patient visit or task the prescriber for follow-up?

- Who is responsible for adding and following through on the information?

  ○ What are the secretary's, nurse's, and prescriber's roles?

  ○ Are these roles different depending on the situation? How?

Historical Prescriptions

Patients take prescription medications, vitamin supplements, herbal remedies, and OTC remedies. E-prescribing uses this information to drive clinical decision support.[71] The more information available, the more valuable the clinical decision support can be.[91] E-prescribing may change workflows for ensuring the medication history is accurate. Offices considering e-prescribing should consider the following:

- What is the primary method for getting medication history information into the e-prescribing application?

○ Automatic medication history may occur through:

- Infrastructure providers such as SureScripts and RxHub

- An integrated health system or HIE initiative

- Pharmacy e-renewal requests (populates over time)

○ Manual medication history entry may be needed when:

- Patients utilize OTC remedies and dietary supplements.

- Patients are not members of the payer and pharmacy networks such as SureScripts, RxHub, and others.

- The e-prescribing application does not support medication history from SureScripts, RxHub, or others.

Reconstituted Histories

Medication histories retrieved from an infrastructure company must be reviewed and edited to be useful. All past medications retrieved in this manner are displayed as active regardless of the patient's actual use. For example, a short-term antibiotic dispensed 3 months ago will appear as active the first time the medication history is retrieved. The prescriber should review the history and take appropriate actions to discontinue medications that have finished their course or are no longer active.

- Who is responsible for entering the patient's medication information and when?

  ○ Will this activity be part of patient check-in, the patient visit, or at checkout?

  ○ Will this trigger other responsibilities such as checking for interactions with other drugs on the patient's profile?

  ○ What level of detail will be required—just the name of the supplement or medication? Are the dose, administration schedule, and manufacturer also needed?

Patient Demographics

New patients come to the office, others leave, some patients move, and others marry; patient demographics need to be maintained. Most demographic changes are managed automatically through an interface with the practice

℞ Pharmacy Perspective

Some pharmacy applications have a difficult time accepting nondispensed medications, though the importance for drug and allergy checking is clear. How can the pharmacist get this information?

- Pharmacists can work with the pharmacy vendor to obtain the same medication history available to the prescribers from the infrastructure providers.

- Pharmacists can investigate acquiring access to medication histories through HIE initiatives and integrated health systems.

- Pharmacists can advise patients to request a current medication list from their prescriber at their next visit.

Pharmacists who have a close business relationship with a prescriber who uses an internet-accessible application can ask to be added as a user. This option is best reserved for pharmacies servicing the entire population of the prescriber or a very well defined population; HIPAA concerns are significant and need to be addressed in this situation. Once the regulatory hurdles are cleared, several advantages emerge, including:

- As a user, the pharmacy can assist in the entry of medication orders directly into the e-prescribing application. This may facilitate e-prescribing implementation for the prescriber.

- The pharmacist can ensure the medications in the e-prescribing application match the drug stock dispensed and that patient instructions are complete, including indications.

- The pharmacy has access to expanded information that may include allergies, complete medication history, and patient problem list.

management system. For those situations requiring manual intervention, the following workflow questions should be considered:

- Who is responsible for patient demographics?
  - Who is responsible for new patients? For changes to existing patients?
  - Who will update the patient's insurance information?
  - Who will update the patient's pharmacy information?
- When will demographics be updated?
  - On check-in?

○ During the visit?

○ After the visit?

E-prescribing adds more to communication options into the office environment. In many cases, the workflow may dramatically change to create new efficiencies. Adapting to these changes takes patience and a high level of communication throughout the implementation process.

Prescribing

Just as e-prescribing introduced new options for communication, it also introduces new ways to generate and manage prescriptions. Translating the complex decisions made by different office staff as they contribute to the management of the prescribing process requires the attention of an astute administrator. The following questions focus on the workflows defining the roles and responsibilities staff carry in relationship to the prescribing process.

Security

E-prescribing has at least two broad security levels: security related to unauthorized application access and, internally, unauthorized application use.

- How many administrators (usually the highest security level of access) will be set up in the application? More administrators translate into less security but more flexibility.

- Staff are hired; staff leave—sometimes with their user names and passwords. What process is used to ensure new users are added in a timely fashion and departing staff have their accounts inactivated?

- Who is responsible for setting and resetting passwords?

- What level of security in the e-prescribing application will be allowed?

  ○ Will the user name/password be the primary security feature for application access?

  ○ Will the administrator require a password for each prescription?

- Will the application automatically log a user out after 5 minutes, 15 minutes, or never?

- What procedure does the administrator have for a suspected security breach?

  ○ Who is notified?

  ○ What patient information might be involved?

    ◦ What is the administrator's responsibility under HIPAA and state privacy laws? (A full discussion of HIPAA requirements including business associate agreements, patient consent, and security is beyond the scope of this book; others such as Hale[38] and Greenberg[26] have covered this area well. Another excellent resource for HIPAA questions is www.hhs.gov/ocr/hipaa/.)

Assistant Prescribing Roles

Robust tools in many e-prescribing applications facilitate the office staff's support of the prescribing process. Unless the prescriber is the only individual using the e-prescribing application, the following workflow issues should be considered:

- Many state laws allow the employee of the physician to relay prescription information to the pharmacy.

  - ◦ What does the state law require? If in doubt, the administrator should do the following:

    - Ask a pharmacist; pharmacists also bear legal responsibility for the prescriptions they dispense and can provide good information as to whether a prescription is legal or not.

    - Check with the local state pharmacy board. A listing of pharmacy boards can be found at: www.edhayes.com/sbp-main.html.

  - ◦ Are forms of indirect authorization such as order sets or standing orders allowed in the office's state?

- If employees are allowed to relay prescriptions, will the nurse or medical office assistant renew prescriptions on behalf of the prescriber? For example, the nurse might renew all pharmacy and patient-requested prescriptions that do not generate an alert or contain an attached note to the contrary.

- If staff are allowed to relay prescriptions, will they preprocess new prescriptions for prescriber final authorization? For example, the nurse generates standard orders for vaccinations and respiratory treatments to be administered in the office, and the prescriber authorizes them at a later time.

- Will prescriptions go to the medical office assistant or nurse for finishing? This process may include printing patient education material, printing labels for samples, and sending the prescription to the pharmacy.

Alerts

Clinical decision support is one of the benefits of e-prescribing. Because the application's capabilities determine the boundaries, a good understanding of the e-prescribing application is needed to answer these workflow questions:

- How will formulary and clinical drug alerts be handled? If the application allows, will the administrator require a reason for overrides on all alerts or only specific categories such as drug allergy alerts or therapeutic duplications?

- How should support staff react to alerts, if displayed?

  ○ Will they be able to override alerts, if the application allows it, or will the order be forwarded to a prescriber for authorization?

  ○ What alerts can be overridden by support staff?

- What will signal the need to adjust alert settings to reduce alert fatigue?

  ○ Will someone review a report of alerts generated and the prescriber's subsequent action?

Physical Layouts

The equipment used in e-prescribing is not as portable as a prescription pad and pen. Accessibility of the equipment may limit implementation in some offices. To understand the degree to which a physical office layout will affect use of e-prescribing technology, office managers should consider these workflow questions.

- How will staff access the e-prescribing application?

  ○ Through PDAs?

  ○ Using desktop computers?

  ○ Via tablets or notebook computers?

- Where will e-prescribing functions take place?

  ○ At the front desk?

  ○ In patient exam rooms? If so, are power supplies available for tablets and notebook computers?

  ○ At workstations?

  ○ In a combination of locations?

- When will prescriptions be written?

  ○ At check-in?

  ○ During the patient visit?

  ○ After the patient visit but before checkout?

- Do all staff who need access to the e-prescribing application have access?

Putting the Patient in the Prescriptive Process

The physical layout of the office determines the level of integration possible with e-prescribing and daily workflow. Users should find a workflow they're comfortable with that also complements their office layout. Though the possibilities are many, here are a few to consider:

- *Focus on Sharing*: The prescriber who focuses on sharing invests in a wireless network and uses a tablet or notebook in patient exam rooms. This allows for sharing and discussion of the patient's medical record as part of the visit along with completion of prescription-related tasks.

- *Focus on Efficiency*: The prescriber focused on efficiency has staff screen for prescription renewals as the patient is checked in. While walking the patient out, the prescriber stops at the central workstation and completes the renewals and new prescriptions. No equipment other than the existing desktop computers and internet access is needed.

- *Focus on Convenience*: The prescriber who focuses on convenience utilizes a PDA during patient visits in place of a prescription pad. Between patient visits, the prescriber stops at the central workstation to authorize staff-processed renewal requests.

Administrative

E-prescribing technology runs on hardware and software. As such, it requires maintenance and administration. In addition to the part played in security, administrators may also have responsibility overseeing the generation of reports from the e-prescribing application.

Helpful Roles

Two roles, the e-prescribing champion and the local expert, if assumed by staff in the office, make implementation easier and more likely to succeed.

Who will be the champion for e-prescribing within the office? This is the person, not necessarily an expert on the e-prescribing application, who motivates the office and gets the staff engaged in the process. The champion is the visionary who clearly sees the potential of the new technology and effectively communicates that vision to others.

(continues)

Helpful Roles *(continued)*

The expert is the internal resource for the office who keeps implementation moving forward. The expert assists in planning for implementation, answers questions unaddressed by training, and troubleshoots problems that come up during implementation. The expert puts legs on the champion's vision.

Reports

Data is one of e-prescribing's assets, and reports mine that data to produce meaningful information. Taking advantage of this information requires consideration of these workflow questions:

- What reports will be printed and how frequently?
- Who will be responsible for printing the reports?
- When will reports be run?
- Who receives the reports, and how do the reports reach their intended audience?
  - Internal mail?
  - E-mail?
- Can the application produce reports that replace existing workflows?
- What is the purpose for generating the report?
  - Is it informational? Such as brand versus generic utilization.
  - Is it regulatory? Such as:
    - The active patient medication list[33]
    - Patients affected by a medication recall; users should consider the recall of Vioxx by Merck[114]
  - Is it for quality assurance? Such as:
  - The daily prescription log
  - Transmission log

Really Useful Reports

One facility created a duplicate of every prescription written, then faxed the medication changes to a community health nurse operating in the field.

(continues)

Really Useful Reports *(continued)*

Personnel at the facility discussed strategies to accomplish this task from the e-prescribing application with the least amount of work possible. At one point in the discussion, someone asked why the prescription was used. The answer, it turned out, was "That's the way we've always done it." What the nurse really needed was information regarding orders changed, added, or discontinued. The e-prescribing application could generate a report by prescriber that did just that for any given time period. This transformed the challenge of getting a prescription to multiple places simultaneously to a workflow procedure in which the secretary generates this report at the end of the day and faxes it to the community health nurses.

Each report carries its own unique workflow considerations with it. For example, if the patient's active medication list is printed before the patient's visit, the prescriber can review it during the visit, but the list will not reflect recent changes. If the list is generated after the visit, it will reflect current changes but may extend the visit time and doesn't give the prescriber a hard copy to work with during the visit.

The information available in the e-prescribing application drives the information on reports. Do workflows provide the data for the desired reports? For example, if a prescriber wants a report on medications prescribed for diabetics, but he doesn't enter diagnoses into the e-prescribing application, his report will be blank.

Attention to the administrative workflow details will support and strengthen the implementation of e-prescribing.

Configuring the E-Prescribing Application

Planning and configuring is a circular process. Once the workflows are identified, the e-prescribing application can be configured to support the workflows. Some workflows work well, and others require retooling to make them fit within the application's capabilities. Security and alerts are some settings the administrator will need to evaluate.

The Circular Nature of Workflows

A prescriber identifies a process within her office for renewal requests. Everyone has a defined role, from the nurse to the receptionist to the prescriber.

(continues)

The Circular Nature of Workflows *(continued)*

But the e-prescribing application doesn't allow the secretary to interact with renewals in the way the prescriber envisions, and the nurse has more access than the prescriber wanted. The prescriber goes back to the workflows and redesigns everyone's role in a manner that accommodates the settings available within the e-prescribing application. Back in the application, the new roles fit well and the prescriber notices the nurse could actually do a little more, something the prescriber hadn't considered before. As a result, she refines the workflows further to take advantage of the e-prescribing functions.

The best workflows are honed and shaped to match the needs of the office within the capabilities of the e-prescribing application in order to fully realize the benefits of e-prescribing.

Configuring Security

The administrator needs to have a good understanding of staff roles and workflows in order to set up user profiles and appropriate security levels.

Configuring Alerts

Another task that falls to the administrator is setting parameters for clinical alerts (see **Table 11.2**). E-prescribing applications frequently have the ability to screen patient profiles for drug interactions, allergy interactions, and more. The clinical alert settings have a profound effect on the experience the users have when actively writing or renewing prescriptions. Setting the sensitivity for the alerts too high will smother the prescriber with warning flags of questionable clinical relevance. Setting the alert sensitivity too low or turning it off entirely will allow dangerous interactions to pass through undetected.

Clinical Alert Dangers

Alert fatigue erodes the effectiveness of clinical decision support; appropriate alert settings are critical. Users should use the application's reports, work with the vendor, and experiment with the application's settings to find a balance they are comfortable with. Determine a priori what conditions are sufficient to readjust the clinical alert settings. This takes some emotional frustration out of implementation. The testing tips in Appendix C can help readers find the right setting.

TABLE 11.2 Alert Settings

Allergy Alerts

Consider—Allergy alerts trigger about 16% of the time with 80% or more overridden. Of those overridden, more than 90% are due to nonexact matches (applying a class effect when none is warranted).[78] The lower trigger rate implies the risk of alert fatigue is less, and, in many cases, the allergy flags can be controlled by judicious entry of allergies into the e-prescribing application. Some applications do have class vs. drug differentiation and wider implementation of this feature appears imminent.

Suggestions—Efforts to improve allergy alerts should be focused on providing alert suppression and differentiating between class-level allergies and specific drug allergies.

Duplicate Therapy Alerts

Consider—Of the alerts triggered, about 61% are due to therapeutic duplication. Since many triggers rely on matching therapies instead of drug families, the utility is widely perceived to be low.[100] Therapeutic duplications are responsible for about 6% of all prescribing errors.[75] This alert has a high trigger rate, low utility, and low contribution to errors. Refinements are needed to increase its utility.

Suggestions—Efforts to improve therapeutic duplication alerts should be focused on providing alert suppression and differentiating between class-level therapies and specific drug families.

Drug Dose Alerts

Consider—Dosing errors account for up to 60% of all prescribing errors.[75] Their trigger rate is relatively low, making the dose alert a valuable option to turn on. In applications that allow further adjustment of this alert for maximum and minimum doses, a further note is warranted. Maximum dose alerts will be more valuable than minimum dose alerts. The minimum alerts may be confounded by the use of half tablets, sample dispensing, and changing therapies, whereas maximum dose alerts typically reflect errors in order entry.

Suggestions—Efforts to improve dose alerts should be focused on increasing the context sensitivity of the alerts with respect to the patient's diagnoses and concomitant medications.

Drug Interaction Alerts

Consider—Drug interaction alerts have the lowest override rate and tend to be more effective than other alerts.[64] Further refinements that help to reduce alert fatigue such as adjusting the display of alerts based on onset level, severity level, and documentation level may be available. Consider a setting of allowing delayed onset since the severity of the reaction is not related to the time of onset. Consider allowing moderate severity interactions to display since many of these can contribute to morbidity; this still avoids a large number of minor interactions. Consider a documentation level of probable to minimize alert fatigue while still capturing reasonable alerts.

No settings will be 100% accurate. After users have some experience with the initial settings, they can make refinements according to their practice.

Suggestions—Efforts to improve drug interactions should be focused on increasing the context sensitivity of the alerts with respect to the dose ordered, the patient's diagnoses, and concomitant medications. Selective alert suppression is also needed.

Learning the e-prescribing application is the easy part; developing new workflows takes time.[18] Defining the new roles and responsibilities prior to e-prescribing implementation contributes significantly to patient safety.

Testing the Workflows

It's important to realize that an e-prescribing application may not support the workflows as fully as the user intended. Users should challenge themselves with actual patient experiences and clinical situations to see how well their workflows work. Consider the following sample situations:

- A patient from another state calls in a panic because a missed flight has caused him to run out of sustained-release oxycodone. Controlled substance prescriptions cannot be transmitted electronically. What steps happen?

- An elderly couple tells a prescriber they are going to Italy for the next 3 months and need a complete set of renewals. How can the prescriber process the renewals for foreign country travel?

- A patient is discharged from the nursing home rehabilitation center and needs 16 medications renewed at her local pharmacy. How are multiple renewals handled?

- A new patient comes to the doctor's office for management of his low back pain. He also receives prescriptions from his cardiologist, endocrinologist, gastroenterologist, urologist, and rheumatologist. How is his profile updated?

- A patient presents with no health insurance but needs multiple samples. How could the prescriber handle this dispensing in the e-prescribing application?

- A resident physician assistant and nurse practitioner rotate through a practice for 8 weeks. How does the administrator set up these users in the application? What level of access do they have?

Training

With newly minted workflows in hand, we turn our attention to training. Adequate training is essential to a successful implementation and continuation of e-prescribing. Of the training types available, competency-based methods are likely to be most successful.[121]

Competency-based training focuses on providing staff with the minimum skill set needed to perform their intended roles. One can tell if training is competency based when the training results in a skill instead of knowledge. That isn't to say that the training imparts no knowledge to the trainee, but that the knowledge gained in a competency-based program is taken to the level of application.

Many vendors' materials convert into a competency-based training program with a little adjusting and ingenuity. The trainer can start with the roles already developed and list the major functions of each role. This defines the functional tasks that need to be performed. Those tasks can be broken down into smaller skills, which can be identified in the vendor's training material. This process also uncovers gaps, if any, in the training material. **Table 11.3** lists examples of skills needed for e-prescribing.

The amount of training per role depends on the number of functions that role needs to perform. Training a secretary responsible only for ensuring

TABLE 11.3 E-Prescribing Skills

Administrators
Application configuration
Clinical alert settings
Managing users

Assistants
Managing emergencies
Managing tasks
New prescriptions
Renewing prescriptions
Basic computer skills
Custom medications
Custom patient instructions (Sig)
Managing allergies
Managing insurance
Managing order favorites
Managing patient demographics
Managing patient problems/procedures list
Managing prescription destinations
Managing reports
Managing the transmission log

Prescribers
Managing emergencies
Managing tasks
New prescriptions
Renewing prescriptions
Safe prescribing habits
Using formularies
Using patient medication history

Finding Skills from Functions

Workflow Function: The nurse processes prescription renewal requests from pharmacies and patients according to the prescriber's direction. Prescriptions are sent to the prescriber for authorization.

Skills Needed

- Sign on and off the application
- Search for and select a patient
- Access the patient's medication history
- Renew a medication
- Identify an alert
- Send a prescription with an alert to the prescriber
- Attach comments to the prescription if necessary
- Print the prescription
- Select a pharmacy
- Send the renewed prescription to the pharmacy
- Cancel a pending prescription

Not all these steps are possible in all e-prescribing applications, but the example serves to illustrate the breakdown of a workflow function into discrete skills. The listing of steps associated with role-defined functions creates the competency checklist. Some skills will be duplicated when other functions are mapped out in this way. This is one of the advantages of the competency-based focus. A skill such as logging on needs to be evaluated by itself. It doesn't matter if the person is logging on to renew a prescription or logging on to print patient education. If the person assuming the nurse role can satisfactorily demonstrate performance of these skills, he can be reasonably expected to function with at least a minimum level of competence wherever those skills are required.

insurance is accurate takes less time than training a secretary responsible for handling renewals, printing prescriptions, printing patient education, and registering patients in the application. Trainers should allow at least an hour for each category of skills—basic skills, prescribing skills, and administrative skills. They should allow an extra hour for practice and development of competency. For example, a prescriber should allow 4 hours for training, 5 if assuming an administrative role. Actual training times will vary according to the aptitude and ability of the person learning.

Four hours for a prescriber is a lot of time to set aside. When an entire office staff needs training, the problem can become a significant scheduling challenge. How will the time for training affect the office workflow? Several options are available for squeezing training time into the office day. If the assessment is done, the office manager will already know what training will work best for her office. If not, **Table 11.4** provides a quick recap.

The assessment discussed in the previous chapter provides guidance as to the best method of training for staff; here is where detail is added to the assessment.

Trainers must give thought to their expectations surrounding e-prescribing training. Unfortunately, many training sessions are summarized as follows: a single date is set, the expert comes, flies through the application, asks for questions, and then disappears. Only a business card with the help line support number is left to flutter in his wake.

An alternative to this cram session is to plan for a staged training approach. Trainers could split the session in two and have the instructor come for the initial training. The rest of the week could be used for staff practice. This allows the trainer to capture the common questions and challenges with the application. The instructor could come back the following week to answer questions, assess competencies, and provide specific training in the areas identified as needing the most support. Generic training sheets in Appendix F could be used to guide training.

In a perfect world, we have the luxury of such planning. In the real world, disruptive events occur regularly, such as staff calling in sick, half the patients getting diarrhea at the same time, or a storm knocking out the electricity on the

TABLE 11.4 Time Shifting Strategies and Costs

Strategy	Cost
Scheduling 25% fewer patients during the training week	Revenue may drop with lower patient volume.
After-hours training	Overtime or additional staff hours might be incurred.
Break training into smaller components that fit into times such as lunchtime, before the office opens, or after the office closes	This is inefficient and may deliver fragmented, inconsistent training.
Reorganize the patient schedule to string together visit slots likely to stay open and use that time for training	The visit slots may suddenly become filled; the method is inherently unpredictable.

day of training. Contingency plans are needed; the office manager should ask the vendor if retraining is available and for how long. Other training considerations include:

- What is the liability if a training date falls through?

- Can the staff sustain intermediate processes in the event the training is delayed?

- Will someone be trained to a higher level so as to train others? The expert is a good candidate for the role of future trainer. Lacking an expert, a champion is another option for a trainer.

Defining Success

Though much of e-prescribing is the application, which the vendor can train the staff to use, the workflow is a significant piece as well; the definition of a successful training should incorporate both of these elements. A competency-based approach assists in creating this definition. Applying the definition to staff on an ongoing basis may identify retraining needs.

The end result of a successful implementation will only be as sound as the least competent staff member. Taking time to ensure everyone achieves the minimum level of competency to function is time well spent on reducing the potential for error that lives in the prescribing process.

Disaster Preparedness

The tyranny of the unknown rules our lives as much as we try to ignore it, though some areas in health care, such as emergency medicine, specialize in the unexpected and unpredictable. How are those emergencies handled? The physician doesn't know an industrial accident will spray acid on six workers. But the emergency department is ready if it does. It has a plan in place. It has the skill to handle it. It has the right equipment ready.

Preparing for a disaster is not about trying to predict what will happen as much as it is controlling the effects of a disaster. In the midst of an emergency, it doesn't matter *why* the power went out, what matters is that work continues *when* the power is out. The reason *why* there's no internet access doesn't provide guidance for handling the patient at the window. Understanding why a disaster happened is interesting, informative, and something that happens retrospectively.

The first step to a successful disaster plan is to take the workflows and assume that whole sections are broken or unavailable. The staff should try to have an alternate plan for each major function in the prescribing process.

Some scenarios to address are:

- Inability to access the e-prescribing application

- Inability to write e-prescriptions

- Inability to renew e-prescriptions

- Inability to add or edit patients

- Inability to print or send to a pharmacy

Paper Prescriptions

It is important to realize that writing paper prescriptions is not easily resurrected as a solution. Writing paper prescriptions, even temporarily, when the office is set up for e-prescribing is different than writing paper prescriptions in a paper-based office. The office using e-prescribing needs to capture prescription information for later entry into the e-prescribing application.

Once a workflow that describes what to do when no one can access the e-prescribing application is in hand, it can be used as the disaster process, the alternative workflow that ensures patients will still receive prescriptions.

The next step is to investigate when the process is implemented. What conditions will trigger the alternative processes? For example, if the alternate process is to use paper prescriptions for a network crash, how long does the network have to be down before the decision is made to switch?

Working backwards from what to when leads us to why. Each disaster scenario generates its own set of questions that are useful in refining the alternate course of action such as environmental difficulties and technical difficulties.

Environmental Difficulties

Disaster such as an ice storm, hurricane, or tornado may challenge the office, as could something as mild as construction down the road severing a power line. Questions to ask include:

- Is the electricity on?

    - If so, can the e-prescribing application still be accessed from other locations such as a home computer, PDA, or cell phone?

    - If not, when will power likely be restored? Is it worth waiting for the power to come back on, or is it better to start handing out paper prescriptions?

- Is prescription data backed up in the event of a catastrophe?
  - Where is it stored?
  - How easy is it to restore the data?
  - Is the pharmacy affected?
    - Should prescriptions be phoned in?
    - Does the fax machine still work?

Technical Difficulties

Sometimes technology doesn't work for reasons often unknown. The lights are on, the sun is shining, and the computer just doesn't work right. In these cases, consider:

- Does the application work at all or are portions of the application simply not responding? If other functions are still working, such as those of a nonprescriber role, can they be used to print prescriptions?

- If the application resides on a server, is there a problem with the connection?

- How long will technical support take to resolve the issue? Is it worth waiting for tech support or should staff use paper prescriptions?

Starting with a strong alternative process that works independent of the reasons why strengthens the disaster process. Incorporating refinements for the why adds depth to the plan. There's an example of a disaster preparedness flowchart in Appendix D.

Half the disaster plan is what is done during the emergency; the other half is how to recover from it. There is also a sample form in Appendix D that can be used as a temporary prescription log. The log is designed to make recovery of prescription information easier than alternative methods of capturing the same information. The prescriptions could be copied on their way out (if the copier works) or written over again; however, recording the essential information on a single log helps minimize the chance of losing a prescription and keeps everything in one place. Also, having a place to indicate if the prescription was entered or not makes it easy to stop and resume the recovery process.

Sample questions aiding in the design recovery process are:

- How will the prescription information be captured?
  - Will a paper log be used?
  - Will copies be handwritten?

- ○ Will the prescription be captured by automated medication history functions or e-renewal requests?

- Who will enter the information during recovery?

- When will prescription information be entered into the e-prescribing application?

- What stress will entering the e-prescriptions place on the office; how does that affect the normal daily work?

Every disaster plan will be unique to the office that creates it, yet many of the elements are similar. Using the above questions and situations as a foundation will assist in constructing a plan that works best for each office. The plan may be simple or complex but most importantly, there is a plan.

Implementation

All the work put into planning pays off in implementation. About 4 to 6 weeks prior to the go-live date for implementation, work should begin on patient demographics and orders. These challenges comprise the lion's share of nonplanning preparatory work. Addressing these issues prior to implementation has a double benefit: office managers complete a critical task and reinforce the e-prescribing training at the same time.

Patient Demographics

Patient information needs to get into the e-prescribing application. At present, there are two ways to get this done: an electronic interface or manual entry.

Electronic Interfaces

The full interface requires an electronic source of patient demographics in order to be an option. Sources of demographic information include a practice management or billing system, an IPA, a large health system, or an HIE. Once installed, the interface transfers the demographics from the source into the e-prescribing application in a manner that is efficient, continuously operating, and (usually) transparent. Those looking for an interface should consider the following options:

- The e-prescribing vendor may have an interface developed. If not, she may be able to direct those who need the interface to someone who does.

- The IT department of a large healthcare system may be able to create an interface, though its interest in doing so may depend on the office's relationship with the system and the software applications being used. The healthcare system will likely be more interested in developing the interface if it is a data source.

- The vendor for the practice management system may be able to develop an interface or direct his clients to someone who can.

- Independent programmers can be contracted to develop an interface, in cooperation with the vendors of the two applications that need to communicate.

A partial interface transfers historical patient information in a single, one-time process. Unlike the continuously operating full interface, the partial interface is used once during implementation and future patient demographics are added directly into the e-prescribing application. Sometimes the source system doesn't communicate directly with the e-prescribing application but it can export to a common file format such as comma separated values (csv) or text (txt), which the application can accept. There are a few reasons to consider a partial interface:

- The patient base is stable and doesn't change much.

- Users need more control over the process, which a common file format affords.

- From a financial perspective, it's the only option within the budget.

- A solid workflow exists for ensuring patients are managed in both applications.

Manual Entry

Entering patients by hand is always an option. Some e-prescribing applications have made this process very streamlined through the use of a reverse-lookup function. The user types in a phone number, and the application searches several databases to fill in the address and city. In most cases, manual entry serves as a supportive feature rather than the primary means of loading demographics.

Users may find a partial interface meets their needs for the initial bulk load while a manual entry process is best to maintain patient information.

Even the best interface or data extraction may have gaps in the patient records, usually due to missing information in the source file. If the patients who cannot be transferred to the e-prescribing application are known, a process to ensure they are added manually can be established. If the patients who cannot be added are unknown, an ongoing process to screen for and enter patients missing in the application can be developed.

Choosing Appropriate Methods

Office managers should keep the big picture in mind when making the decision between manual entry and interfaces. One office's total patient population was less than 350. For them, entering the patients manually (it was a stable population) was the most expedient option.

Patient Medication History

Getting patient demographics into the e-prescribing application is the easy task. The greater challenge is populating the patient's profile with current medications. Thankfully, technology is available to make this process as painless as possible (see Chapters 2 and 3). In the absence of infrastructure providers such as SureScripts or RxHub, importing medication information from other sources usually requires multiple interfaces. Whether users will be able to take advantage of the technology depends on the application they are using. As time passes, solutions to this obstacle should become more common. Until then, a few points require discussion.

There is rarely a good, complete source of patient medications. The insurance company has one piece, the pharmacy another, the healthcare application another, the physician another, and the patient still another. It can be amazingly difficult to differentiate the medications a given patient is supposed to be taking as opposed to what he is actually taking. This places even greater importance on the e-prescribing application as a repository of the current medication list. See also Chapter 6.

Medications: Missing, Mythical, and Mistaken

Much of the difficulty in constructing an accurate medication list is the result of a perfect storm of technological limitations, human inconsistency, and communication challenges.

- *Technological Limitations*: Some pharmacy programs cannot accommodate entry of nondispensed or OTC medications. Insurance companies

(continues)

Medications: Missing, Mythical, and Mistaken *(continued)*

have difficulty capturing OTC medications and medications for which they do not pay. Physician records suffer inconsistencies in documentation of OTCs and medications ordered by other specialists. Most patients don't have a technological means of tracking their medications.

- *Human Inconsistencies*: Patients may decide to stop taking a medication or alter the dose on their own. Documentation in medical offices and pharmacies may be inconsistent. Patient medication lists may not be updated and patients may misremember medications they take.

- *Communication Challenges*: There is no easy way to compare records across patient, insurer, pharmacy, and prescriber. E-prescribing is making some headway, but there's no way to determine which information takes precedence. The names of medications are complex and difficult for many patients to pronounce, resulting in errors when generating a medication list from an oral history.

Entering medication orders takes time. Regardless of the amount of technological aid, there is a significant degree of manual entry during the implementation period. Planning is required to allow staff time to get medication histories entered. The assessment discussed in Chapter 10 touched on this briefly, and now we'll explore the options in more detail.

Medication histories are available from RxHub and SureScripts, which, if the application can take advantage of the technology, will greatly reduce the time needed to get patient profiles current. Even so, the manual process is needed to fill in the gaps. There are three methods for updating medication histories that can be combined to meet the office needs—front loading, back loading, and as-you-go training. **Table 11.5** compares these three approaches.

Office managers should consider prioritizing the medication history entry with a method that best meets the office's needs. There are three main focus areas that could be considered, as follows:

- *Focus on Acuity*: These are the patients seen every 3 months; their charts are measured in inches and pounds. The likelihood of a hospital admission is greatest in this population, and, by extension, the benefit of a complete electronic medication history is greater as well.

- *Focus on Schedule*: Users should look forward in the schedule to the next week or two and ensure patients who have appointments scheduled during that time have accurate medication histories in the application.

- *Focus on Order*: An alphabetical or other structured approach may meet the office needs.

TABLE 11.5 Loading Medication Histories

The Front Loader

The bulk of the medication history is downloaded or entered prior to the go-live date.

Advantages
- Staff gain experience and can troubleshoot the most common problems prior to going live.
- Operational slowdowns due to data entry are more easily controlled prior to going live.
- Safety. High-risk patients are entered, and if hospitalization occurs before their visit, the med list is in an electronic form.
- Relatively quick conversion of med profiles to electronic form.

Disadvantages
- Operations may slow as staff absorb the additional burden of prescription entry.
- Creates an additional workflow process.

Example Methods
- Patient schedules for the next 3 months are printed.
- Identify patients on the schedule list taking significant (four or more) number of medications.
- Staff with limited to full prescribing authority trigger medication history downloads or enter the current medication profiles into the Rx program. (Staff with limited authority will still need prescriptions verified by those with full authority.)
- Other patients are entered into the application as they come in.

As You Go

The bulk of the medication history is downloaded or entered after the go-live date as patients come into the office.

Advantages
- Efficiency. Entry is done as patients come in—this is the most efficient use of prescriber time.
- May be more accurate if done just after or during a patient visit.
- May be the easiest process to insert into normal operations.

Disadvantages
- Overall conversion of med profiles may be protracted.
- Lengthens the workday for several months.
- May affect visit turnaround time.
- Decreased ability to troubleshoot, especially retrospectively. Increased acuity of troubleshooting needs due to time constraints.
- Medication list may be incomplete for at least a year.

Example Methods
- Patient schedules for the current day are printed.
- Staff with limited to full prescribing authority trigger medication history downloads or enter the current medication profiles into the Rx program. (Staff with limited authority will still need prescriptions verified by those with full authority.)

The Back Loader

The bulk of the medication history is downloaded or entered after the go-live date after the business day is done.

Advantages
- Flexible time—entry is done outside the workflows of the office.
- Flexible approach—can choose to enter prospectively (using printed schedules of future visits) or retrospectively (past visits).

continues

TABLE 11.5 *(continued)*

Disadvantages
- Conversion of med profiles may be modestly protracted.
- Lengthens the work day for several months.
- Decreased ability to troubleshoot, especially retrospectively.
- May result in greatest demands on prescriber's time.
- Medication list is incomplete for at least a year.

Example Methods
- Patient schedules for the current day or for future visits are printed.
- Staff with limited to full prescribing authority trigger medication history downloads or enter the current medication profiles into the e-Rx program. (Staff with limited authority will still need prescriptions verified by those with full authority.)

Many offices employ a blended approach, front loading acute patients and using the schedule for the remainder. Regardless of method, proactively addressing medication histories in a structured fashion may provide the greatest benefit for the least amount of energy.

Activities during Implementation

Notification

One of the more exciting tasks is notifying patients and pharmacies of connectivity. Notification has several benefits worth considering:

- The pharmacists may be able to work with the medical office to troubleshoot any issues that surface as a result of implementation. Surescripts has a great resource for sharing connectivity at www.surescripts.com/pdf/PhysicianConnectedLetter.pdf.

- Instilling realistic expectations of e-prescribing into patients provides a cushion of understanding during the sensitive period of implementation and improves acceptance of the technology.

  - E-prescriptions may still experience delays in transmission.

  - E-prescribing does not eliminate delays in the pharmacy that occur from insurance questions, clinical concerns, or prescription volume.

Implementation-Specific Workflows

Certain workflows are temporary, bridging practices that facilitate the implementation process. For example, a change log helps to capture problems encountered during the application's early use. Not only does the change log provide a means of communication with the rest of the users, but it organizes the problems and enhancement suggestions in a form that helps the vendor to work on resolutions. From a supervisor's perspective, the change log reduces the number of duplicate complaints from staff and makes distributing solutions easier. The supervisor should consider posting the change log in a conspicuous location or saving it to a common folder on a computer network. Taking time to discuss the change log is a good practice, even if only to note the absence of recent changes during the weeks of implementation.

Pharmacist Perspective

A change log is a good idea in the pharmacy as well. Other pharmacy application functions may be affected when e-prescribing comes on line.

A plan to address critical failures is essential for maintaining smooth operations. Something will happen—a lost password, a moment's forgetfulness, an application failure—and e-prescribing won't be able to be used. Without a plan to manage this temporary disruption, staff and patients may become frustrated and patient care delayed. Give consideration to an alternate workflow to ensure seamless care. **Table 11.6** lists strategies and suggestions to address this type of disruption. Post help resources prominently around the fax machine, printers, and computers to remind people of the correct process to follow.

Conclusion

Implementation needs vary from office to office; prior planning prevents poor performance. Creating new workflows that use e-prescribing in the most

TABLE 11.6 Temporary Application Problems

Identify a go-to person such as the expert to handle e-prescribing issues.

Script staff responses in a manner that promotes confidence of patients. For example: Instead of "The new program isn't working again," consider "Let me get the doctor to write those prescriptions for you." If pressed, the staff person can respond with something like, "We're still getting used to the new program, but that won't prevent me from caring for you."

Have materials and supplies for the alternate process at hand.

Communicate to staff that the alternate process is not the preferred process.

Utilize an alternate communication convention such as stickies, colored flags, e-mail, or voice mail to communicate e-Rx needs.

Expecting the Unexpected

Challenge: The nurse finds herself locked out; the application doesn't accept her password. She prepares a paper prescription, notes the order for later entry, and leaves a message for the office manager to troubleshoot the problem.

Benefit: Rather than stopping the normal routine to deal with the password, the patient is handled through an alternate process while the e-prescribing issue is resolved behind the scenes.

---

efficient manner for the office is harder than learning the application itself. After implementation is complete, the same process can be used to incorporate each subsequent change in the e-prescribing application into workflows.

The result of this hard work is the union of application and workflow, custom fitted for each office. After the twin hurdles of patient demographics and medication history are cleared, the rest is downhill; maintaining workflows through an ongoing quality assurance process is still needed, but it is less work.

Chapter 12

How to Evaluate E-Prescribing Outcomes

READING PRIORITY

Measuring Outcomes

Today's evidence-based healthcare environment relies on data to propel it forward. E-prescribing places a wealth of data regarding prescribing habits within reach. Currently, outcomes data regarding e-prescribing in primary care offices is minimal at best. Planning for and automating ways to capture and analyze data benefits the medical community as a whole and the office in particular. Potential office benefits listed in **Table 12.1** depend on the specific situation and practice environment. The list is not comprehensive; other benefits may be discovered in activities such as research and teaching.

The process of data collection should be automated as much as possible to minimize work. The following questions aid in designing an optimal outcomes measurement process.

- What are the relevant outcomes for the office? For example, one office may focus on operational efficiencies to justify its return on investment, another focuses on safety measures, and a third focuses on quality measures.

TABLE 12.1 Potential Benefits of E-Prescribing Outcomes Data

Enhanced practice image—Producing data related to patient care is a respectable accomplishment that demonstrates initiative and a commitment to improvement.

Improved patient recruitment and retention—E-prescribing is a tool that differentiates competitors. But what if competitors are e-prescribing as well? Outcomes data becomes the tipping point.

Referrals from peers—Outcomes data makes the good work of a practice visible to others.

Insurer benefits—Outcomes data may make an office stronger against audits. Also, some insurers may offer discounts based on e-prescribing or the ability to demonstrate improved benefits.

Malpractice savings—Some providers of medical malpractice insurance offer a discount if e-prescribing is implemented.

Continuing improvement—One of the most important benefits from outcomes data is the information it provides for improving current systems in an ongoing fashion.

- What measurable variables best represent safety, quality, and operational outcomes? For example, tracking the number of alerts generated by an e-prescribing application may reflect a safety outcome, as does tracking the number of emergency department admissions.

- What data is already captured by existing applications? For example, a decrease in call volume into and out of the office may be measured by the phone system and faxed reports.

- Is the data is accessible? For example, some applications produce a report that is exportable to a common file format while other applications require a custom report to be written, and still others have data that is simply inaccessible.

The ultimate goal of outcomes monitoring is to use the data in a way that improves operations, patient safety, and quality of care. As such, prescribers should consider actions to be taken in the event of positive, negative, or neutral results. What actions will be taken as a consequence of the results?

Data Sources

The phone, fax, and e-prescribing application may serve as data sources within the office while pharmacies, payers, independent practice associations, and patients can be explored as external data sources.

Phones and Faxes

Incoming and outgoing call and fax volume is useful as a before and after comparison since pharmacy-related issues are responsible for many calls and faxes in a medical office. Tracking this information measures the degree to which e-prescribing has shifted communication into the electronic environment. If there isn't a significant change, dialogue with the pharmacies may be required to ensure they are communicating electronically. The reduction in call volume may justify decreasing the number of incoming phone lines—a potential cost-saving benefit.

Average hold time and dropped calls are customer service variables that may improve with the implementation of e-prescribing. Clearing out pharmacy-related calls creates time for patients and other physician offices. If this was a significant problem that is resolved after e-prescribing implementation, prescribers may regain lost business by communicating the improvement to patients and other physician offices.

The amount of office supplies consumed can be measured. A drop in fax volume reduces the need for paper and toner supplies. Office managers can follow the line item for office supply expenses before and after e-prescribing.

Pharmacist Perspective

The pharmacy can track interactive voice response system (IVRS) load. A shift from IVRS to e-prescriptions represents an increase in safety for patients. Physicians with e-prescribing who still use IVRS heavily may benefit from supportive education about electronic prescribing.

E-Prescribing Application Data

The ability of e-prescribing applications to generate usable data varies according to the application. Many of the following suggestions will not be possible with an application's current configuration, will require additional expense, will be available on request from the vendor, or will have the feature built in.

Alerts Triggered

Clinical alert settings determine which alerts are triggered. A report on the type and frequency of alerts can be used to adjust the clinical alert settings so that alerts are optimized. Trending alert frequency is one way to document improved prescribing habits and patient safety.

Alerts Overridden

The reason why an alert is overridden reflects the impact e-prescribing has on patient safety as well as highlighting problematic prescriptions. If the application allows, prescribers should review the reasons alerts are overridden on an ongoing basis. Perhaps an order for enoxaparin always flags an alert with low-dose aspirin inappropriately, indicating a need to suppress that alert. Perhaps an order is flagged as a result of an insurance formulary preference such as using gemfibrozil in place of fenofibrate. Documentation that the insurer's preferred agent consistently generates more alerts than the medication normally prescribed may be useful when justifying a preferred therapy.

Understanding the reasons why alerts are overridden is also valuable for new prescribers joining the practice, and it facilitates their integration into the office. Office prescribing norms are made more visible when reasons for overriding alerts is transparent.

Alerts Resulting in an Order Change

This enhanced report describes what orders are consistently changed and why. Are allergy interactions responsible for most changes? Formulary alerts? Drug interactions? Can this information be used to adjust prescribing habits in a way that reduces the alerts in the future?

Formulary Adherence

This report displays the distribution of prescribing habits against a plan's formulary. In the case of a 3-tiered formulary, the report displays medications prescribed sorted by tier. This can be a useful tool, especially for insurance programs that have a large number of a prescriber's patients as members. Prescribing should be cost effective for patients. Patients tend to be more adherent when their medications are affordable.

Preferred Therapeutic Agents

This report displays the most common prescriptions and provides indirect information about the agents used most frequently to treat a particular diagnosis. This can answer the question, "What antihypertensive do I prescribe most often?"

Prescription Volume Trending

If a prescriber wants to determine if he is writing more prescriptions for a particular drug, or if he wants to prove to himself that pharmaceutical company representatives don't influence his prescribing, he can run a report that shows volume trending. This report can show whether his prescribing is on track with standards when the Food and Drug Administration releases a new black box warning or the Centers for Disease Control releases new guidelines.

Patient Adherence

As medication histories mature, the abilities of this report will expand. Most e-prescribing applications have the ability to pull medication history from infrastructure providers (see also Chapter 2) or through direct relationships with other history sources. This information usually represents what the pharmacy records as a purchase or what the payer is reimbursed for. Matching what was dispensed with the prescription information in the prescriber's application (what was written) generates a picture of the patient's adherence.

Pharmacy Renewals

Sometimes a prescriber wants to know which pharmacies are sending e-renewals, whether there are there problems with a particular pharmacy, or how many renewals from pharmacies he is receiving. The pharmacy renewal report focuses on issues surrounding e-renewals and, if necessary, can provide the documentation needed to approach the pharmacy. Sometimes a small adjustment in the software applications is needed to resolve these issues.

Active Problems

For e-prescribing applications that support an active problem list, compiling a frequency distribution of the diagnoses or problems treated helps to identify shifts in patient demographics and acuity. The e-prescribing application complements the practice management system by reporting on problems for which a prescriber has written prescriptions. This is a different view than the practice management application, which may report on all problems.

Combining problems with prescriptions also allows for identification of conditions responsible for the majority of prescriptions. A prescriber might also be able to determine if the number of medications prescribed for the elderly (adding age into the report) could be reduced, or whether depressed patients use a lot of opiates.

Favorites (Common Orders)

Weeding out unused favorite orders or deleting the entire list should be done at regular intervals, such as quarterly.

> ### ℞ Pharmacist Perspective
>
> Many of these reports are already available within pharmacy applications. In addition, pharmacies can measure the number of will calls and average customer wait time before and after e-prescribing implementation.

Patients, Pharmacies, and Payers

Patients and pharmacies can provide outcome data for prescribers in the form of satisfaction surveys. Other outcomes such as safety and quality can be explored with the combination of patient charts and e-prescribing reports.[39,124] Frequency of drug interaction alerts can be cross-matched with the incidence for drug-related emergency department admissions.

Pharmacies can be a wealth of information for outcomes data as well, depending on the level of cooperation and technical sophistication the prescriber wishes to pursue. For example, pharmacy applications can provide information on patient adherence. Pharmacies can help determine whether patients with e-prescriptions get them filled more often than those with paper prescriptions.

Payers sometimes provide outcomes data in the form of report cards or other measurement tools. These payer-generated reports represent a gold mine of information for understanding the effects of e-prescribing on the prescriber's office. A prescriber might be wondering whether her prescribing has moved closer to standards. She might be asking herself if she is making better therapeutic choices when prescribing. The payer feedback indirectly provides a partial answer to these questions.

Case Studies

The Medical Office

This is a composite case based on experiences in a variety of settings. A busy internal medicine practice with two physicians was looking for ways to attract a third partner. The recent loss of a part-time physician had overloaded the current office's capacity. Most local pharmacies used e-prescribing, and adopting the technology was believed to aid recruitment efforts while decreasing workload. The office manager wanted to know how e-prescribing outcomes should be measured and reported to represent a meaningful attraction to prospective physicians and staff.

What options were available? Information related to the implementation could be gathered into groupings of operational, safety, and quality measures.

Operational measures relate to efficiency, return on investment, and the effect e-prescribing has on business capacity. Safety measures affect the relative safety benefit provided to patients. All safety is quality but not all quality is safety. Quality measures reflect the quality of care and customer service patients receive. The office compiled a list of potential variables to measure in each of these categories.

Operational Measures

- **Phone volume (the number of calls)**
- Phone time (the amount of time spent on the phone per hour)
- Fax volume (the number of faxes)
- Fax time (the amount of time spent transmitting or receiving faxes)
- **Average new prescription processing time**
- **Average prescription renewal processing time**
- Average prescription processing time in detail (split by operator: physician, nurse, secretary; and type: fax, e-script, phone, paper)
- Monthly office supply line-item expense
- Number of prescriptions written per day and per week

Safety Measures

- Number of pharmacy callbacks
- Number and type of alerts triggered
- Number of medications changed due to alerts
- **Number of hospital admissions**
- **Length of work day for secretary, nurse, and physician**
- Number of patients receiving written medication list at visit
- Number of patients receiving written information with samples

Quality Measures

- Average phone hold time
- Amount of generic use

- Number of dropped calls
- **Average patient wait time for visit**
- Average time for ad hoc patient appointment
- **Patient satisfaction survey results**
- **Staff satisfaction survey results**
- Number of failed e-prescribing transmissions

The office manager chose to narrow the list to select operational and quality measures. Using the narrowed list, the staff designed and implemented a plan for outcomes monitoring starting 1 month prior to implementing e-prescribing and continuing for 3 months after implementation. The phone company provided a detailed bill that shows phone and fax line activity. The staff hands out patient surveys with each visit as part of the checkout process. All staff completed a satisfaction survey before implementation, 2 weeks after implementation, and at the end of 4 months. The office manager calculated patient wait time for 10 random patients, tallied the number of patients newly admitted to the hospital, and tracked staff hours worked each week. The patient wait time was based on each patient's sign-in, the appointment time, the time the nurse brought the patient to the exam room, and the time the physician came to the room.

Four months later, the office demonstrated a decrease in prescription processing time and improved satisfaction for patients and staff. Hospitalizations tended to be fewer but more time and events were needed to determine a true difference. Though initially perceived as burdensome, the staff found that e-prescribing lightened the workload 3 months after implementation.

The Pharmacy

This is a composite case based on experiences in a variety of settings. An independent pharmacy serves surrounding physicians and a large healthcare system. A significant number of local physicians were using e-prescribing and the pharmacy was in the process of acquiring the ability to receive e-prescriptions. The pharmacy's administration wanted to know the return on investment and left it to the supervising pharmacist to demonstrate the value of the upgrade to the pharmacy system.

Operational Measures and Operational Capacity

One of the benefits of e-prescribing is a decrease in workload. But personnel costs are a fixed expenditure and attaching a hard dollar value to this benefit is difficult. Using operational capacity helps to recast this value in a manner similar to cost avoidance measures. For example, let's assume a single pharmacist with a technician can reasonably process a maximum of thirty-five prescriptions in an hour or 280 prescriptions in an 8-hour day. This operational capacity is theoretical and may be greater than actual prescription volume. Surges in volume beyond the operational capacity are predictably associated with a marked increase in errors and employee dissatisfaction.

If e-prescribing creates efficiencies that reset the operational capacity to 40 prescriptions an hour or 320 prescriptions daily, that's a 14% increase in efficiency. Business can comfortably grow and operate at a higher volume without requiring the addition of new staff. In effect, expansion of operational capacity has resulted in cost avoidance. The value of operational capacity is not expressed in pharmacist hours saved but in potential revenue gained. If the average revenue per prescription is $40, then the expansion of operational capacity is an increase in revenue capacity of $1,600/day with existing staff.

Operational Measures

- Phone volume (the number of calls)
- Phone time (the amount of time spent on the phone per hour)
- Fax volume (the number of faxes)
- Fax time (the time is spent transmitting or receiving faxes)
- **Average prescription processing time**
- Average prescription processing time in detail (split by operator: technician, RPh; and type: fax, e-script, phone, IVRS, paper)
- **Operational capacity**
- IVRS volume
- **Monthly office supply line-item expense**
- Inventory value
- Sales receipts
- Prescription volume

Safety Measures

- Number of problem prescriptions
- **Outgoing phone volume**

- Number and type of patient interventions
- Patient adherence (prescriptions refilled on time)
- Error tracking results (subset of problem prescriptions)
- Clinical alert frequency

Quality Measures

- Average phone hold time
- **Average customer wait time for prescription**
- **Customer satisfaction survey results**
- Staff satisfaction survey

The pharmacist decided on select operational measures, drafted workflows that addressed ongoing data collection, and created a plan for e-prescribing implementation that included staff training and the newly developed workflows. After 2 weeks of preimplementation monitoring, data was gathered for an additional 3 months. At that time, measurements of prescription processing time yielded an estimated operational capacity increase of about 10%; outbound calls had decreased along with the average customer wait time.

Conclusion

Electronic prescribing is a wonderful tool still in its infancy. An old proverb states, "It takes a village to raise a child," and the adage is true of e-prescribing as well. This technology requires the involvement and cooperation of multiple disciplines.[17] All facets of the healthcare industry are needed to bring e-prescribing technology to its full potential.

Everyone is a patient at one time or another; as such, we all have a vested interest in the way e-prescribing affects safety within health care.

A Model of Error

A Concept of Medication System Safety

The importance of prescription safety cannot be understated in today's healthcare environment. If this discussion began with an attempt to answer the question, "What is an error?" this book would be many chapters longer. As Woods and Cook note in their article, "Mistaking Error," finding a definition for error becomes more elusive the closer one looks.[125]

Definitions of error are useful when measurement is required,[46,101] but they lose their utility when applied to error prevention. If error prevention is effective, there is nothing to measure. This is a major challenge confronting studies that measure error. Was the intervention effective, or was the measuring tool not sensitive enough?

Rather than looking at error directly, let's examine the capacity of systems to produce error. The systems we work with are burgeoning with the potential for error. A hospital is a system. A medical office is a system. E-prescribing is a system. Understanding how a system can fail is half the battle. Doing something about it is the other half. Ritzel, in a fine article covering occupational safety definitions and concepts, suggests that actively reducing the opportunity for error results in a decrease in actual errors.[126]

A ball on the edge of a table can be described by its potential energy. The ball is at rest. All the ball needs is a gentle nudge for gravity, resistance, and mass to convert the potential energy into kinetic energy, putting the ball in motion. In the same way, the systems we work in can be described by the potential for error within them. When the system is in motion, the potential for error changes into actual errors.

For the sake of illustration, the term *hazard estimate* will be used as a quality of a system at rest. The ball, table, floor, and air all represent pieces of a system. The qualities of those components and their relationships to each other all contribute to the expected outcome of a ball falling when it reaches the table's edge. The hazard estimate summarizes the qualities of a system from a safety perspective.

Sometimes a mathematical relationship makes an idea easier to understand. These expressions are for illustration of concepts only and are greatly simplified. The mathematical expression that expresses the hazard estimate might look something like this:

Hazard estimate = Number of subsystems/average communication index

Average communication index is a proxy for the quantity and quality of communication that occurs between two systems. A value of 1 is equal to perfect communication, 0.5 represents no communication, and 0.01 represents misinformation.

This makes intuitive sense. The relative safety of a system is related to the number of subsystems involved and how well those subsystems communicate with each other.[127] As the number of subsystems increases, the relative safety of a system decreases. Likewise, safety declines as communication between subsystems falls. **Figure A.1** provides a graphical example of the larger process that treats the hospital and pharmacy as subsystems of the healthcare system.

If the hazard estimate describes a system at rest, as if laid out on an examination table, what happens when we breathe life into it? What happens when people, information, and equipment start moving through the system? Systems in motion interact with other systems through their boundaries, and

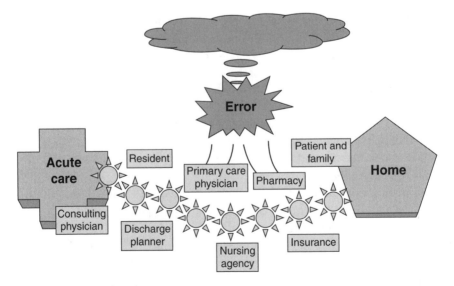

FIGURE A.1 Hazard Ratio

boundaries are where the potential for error is greatest. Tam and colleagues[128] and Flabouris and colleagues[129] provide studies that demonstrate this well.

Let's go back to the ball analogy for a moment. The ball's potential energy increases as the height of the table increases; the potential error a patient is exposed to increases as the hazard estimate of a system increases. If we were to express the potential error as a mathematical equation, it could look like:

$$\text{Potential error (PE)} = \frac{(\text{Hazard estimate} \times \text{boundaries crossed} \times \text{boundary distance})}{(\text{average communication index} \times \text{time of transition})}$$

The term *boundaries crossed* describes the transitions from place to place and from department to department that a patient experiences when moving through healthcare systems. We cross boundaries daily. For example, walking outside the house is crossing a boundary, getting in the car is another, and walking into the building at work is crossing another.

Boundary distance describes the relationship boundaries have with respect to each other. For the sake of illustration, set a value of 1 for separate boundaries, 0.5 for joined boundaries, and 0.1 for overlapped boundaries. In the above example, work is far from home—a separated boundary. If work was joined to home, the door that allows exit from the house is the same door that leads into work—the boundary is joined. But what about work done from home? This involves overlapping boundaries.

Time of transition reflects the constraints imposed by time on this journey. How fast does one travel through the boundaries? To continue the above example, cutting the time it takes to drive to work in half increases the risk of an accident. Time is a variable that helps describe the degree of stress on the systems. In this sense, time is a variable that places a cap on the amount of communication that can occur between systems when crossing a boundary. It is important to note that within a system, the amount of time spent in hazardous processes (such as the amount of time a patient is open on the operating table) should be minimized. The equation describes the transition between systems where longer transitional times are desirable. For example, the hospital discharge process can begin on the day of admission.

This is an overly simplified diagram of very complex processes, but it helps to focus on important concepts. See the comprehensive work done in six sigma systems and healthcare safety for a more detailed discussion of this topic.[130]

If one travels rapidly through a large number of systems that provide misinformation to each other, an error is guaranteed. When many system boundaries are crossed at one time, the potential error increases. If communication between systems is poor, the potential error increases. If the time spent crossing the system boundaries is very short, the potential error increases. One of the best places to see potential error in action is during the typical hospital discharge.

Table A.1 lists common internal systems involved in a hospital discharge, and **Table A.2** refers to those boundaries that can be crossed during discharge.

Now, place this complexity that is internal to the hospital in the context of other systems the patient encounters outside the hospital system, each with its own set of internal complexities (see **Table A.3**).

In a graphical fashion, it is easier to imagine the path of the patient in **Figure A.2** where multiple system boundaries are crossed.

These two concepts, that risk increases as system boundaries are crossed and that safety is a function of the how well a system's components communicate, are essential when discussing electronic prescribing and safety. Prescribing, by its nature, involves, at a minimum, the patient, prescriber, and

TABLE A.1 Examples of Systems Involved in a Hospital Discharge

Department of medicine
Nursing
Radiology
Food services
Environmental services
Social work
Pharmacy
Medical records
Laboratory services

TABLE A.2 Examples of Boundaries That Can Be Crossed During a Hospital Discharge

Shift change
Department routines
Patient mealtimes
Surgery schedule
Staff break times
Discharge procedures
Discharge planning
Patient emergencies
Staffing changes (sick calls, preference)

TABLE A.3 Systems the Patient Encounters Outside the Hospital

Pharmacy
Primary care office
Home health agency
Family
Transportation
Outpatient laboratory
Specialist office

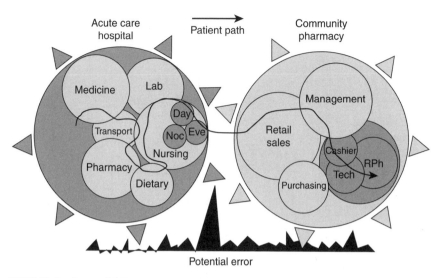

FIGURE A.2 Potential Error

pharmacist. Insurance companies, medical office staff, family members, social agencies, and pharmacy staff add more complexity to this process.

In general, safety is improved when communication is enhanced either by the addition of relevant information into the system or through enhanced access to existing information.[91] Conversely, the potential for error is increased when additional steps are inserted into a process within a system or when the processes themselves are unsound and prone to failure.

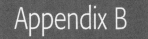

Prior Authorization Fax Tool

_____ **Prior authorization required**
_____ **Nonformulary issue**

_____ **MD office/name**
_____ **MD fax no.**

To expedite patient care, please respond by faxing or calling pharmacy when prior authorization is received.

☐ Please change medication as noted in comments.

Pharmacy contact information	Rx insurance: _____ Insurance ID No.: _____ Rx Insurance Phone No.: _____ Pharmacy screen print attached: Yes ☐ No ☐

Rx label	**Prescriber response: (Check one)** ☐ Prior authorization obtained ☐ Prior authorization pending If applicable, Prior Auth. No.: _____

Please fax or call this prescription change to the pharmacy directly.
Comments:

_____
_____
_____

©2006 Joint Physician Pharmacy Group. A subgroup of the Pharmacy Society of Rochester and the Monroe County Medical Society. Contact: Michael Van Ornum, Chair: Jppg@mac.com; http://homepage.mac.com/mvanornum.

Testing Tips for E-Prescribing Applications

Function	Test	What It Does
Searching	asp	Evaluates combination-partial search for aspirin.
	asp 325	Evaluates partial-letter search for aspirin 325 mg.
	rin 25	Evaluates complex combined partial search for aspirin 325 mg.
	asa	Evaluates recognition of vernacular abbreviations for aspirin.
	Sitagliptin	Evaluates ability to search by generic name when no generic exists. Sitagliptin is the generic name of Januvia.
Results display	Ciprofloxacin Gentamicin Hydrocortisone	Evaluates handling of multiple doses and formulations. Is the display clear? Are the medications well differentiated?

Function	Test	What It Does
	Warfarin 2 mg alternating with 1 mg every other day by mouth to prevent clots. Dispense 30 refill x5.	Requires two separate orders even though it may be written on paper as one order.
	Aspirin 81 mg once daily by mouth to prevent heart attack.	OTC medication
	Albuterol MDI two puffs every 4 hours as needed for asthma. Dispense 3 refill x5.	PRN medication
	Oxycodone 20 mg twice daily by mouth for pain. Dispense 60.	Test alternatives. CII prescription—can't be sent electronically
Prescribing sample orders	Zolpidem 10 mg before bed as needed by mouth for insomnia.	CIV prescription—can't be sent electronically
	Pilocarpine 0.5% two drops to left eye three times daily for glaucoma. Dispense 1 refill x5.	Eye drops
	Calcium + D 600 mg twice daily with meals by mouth to protect bones.	Test interaction with levothyroxine.
	Erythromycin 500 mg three times daily by mouth for URI.	Test interaction with warfarin.
	Omeprazole 20 mg 1 cap daily for GERD. Dispense 30, refill x5 DAW.	Test formulary status.
	Oxygen 2 L via nasal cannula when asleep.	Test nondrug order capability.

Function	Test	What It Does
Dose checking	Acetaminophen 8 gm Q4H PRN.	Test detection of overdoses.
Formulary status	Felodipine 10 mg daily. Felodipine 10 mg daily DAW.	Do both orders produce the same formulary status indicator?
Dosing units	Enoxaparin 40 mg once daily subcutaneously to prevent clots. Dispense 10 refill x1. Lindane shampoo 1% to scalp. Dispense 30 ml refill 0. Hydrocortisone 2.5% cream to affected area twice daily. Dispense 50 gm refill 0. Albuterol 0.083% 3 ml via nebulizer Q2H PRN.	May require a specialty pharmacy. Observe dosing calculator. Observe dosing calculator and dosing units used.
Patient instructions	Alendronate 70 mg. Take once weekly in an upright position at least 1 hour before the first meal of the day and with a full glass of water. Varenicline starting month. Take 0.5 mg once daily for days 1 through 3, then 0.5 mg twice daily for days 4 through 7, then 1 mg twice daily.	Evaluate complex patient instructions.
Cross-platform behavior	Add new patient Add new allergy Add new prescription Send Rx to pharmacy Send Rx to printer Renew Rx Resolve DUR alert	Perform these tasks on each device or environment to evaluate differences in implementation across different devices and environments.

Testing DUR Interactions				
First Drug	Second Drug	Onset	Severity	Documentation
Warfarin	Sertraline	Delayed	Moderate	Fair
Warfarin	Alfalfa	Delayed	Minor	Fair
Warfarin	Gemfibrozil	Delayed	Moderate	Good
Warfarin	Simvastatin	Delayed	Moderate	Excellent
Warfarin	Low molecular weight heparin	Not specified	Major	Fair
Warfarin	Aspirin	Delayed	Major	Excellent
Warfarin	Fenofibrate	Delayed	Major	Good
Sulfamethaxazole and trimethoprim	Pentamidine	Not specified	Major	Fair
Sulfamethaxazole and trimethoprim	Isradipine	Not specified	Major	Fair
Sulfamethaxazole and trimethoprim	Lamivudine	Delayed	Minor	Good

Disaster Preparedness

Figure D.1 depicts a flowchart to aid in managing prescriptions during an emergency.

Figure D.2 provides a sample form that can be used to record prescriptions for later entry into the e-prescribing application in the event of an emergency.

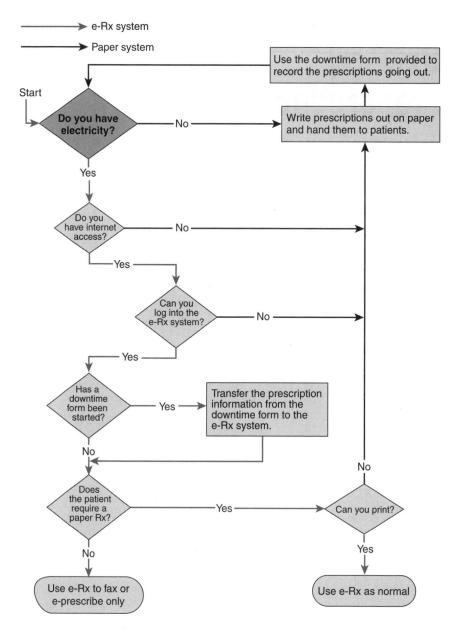

FIGURE D.1 E-Prescribing During an Emergency

Temporary Prescription Log

Date Written	Pt. Name	Prescriber	Medication	Strength	Directions	Quantity	Refills	Pharmacy	Date in E-Rx	Initials

Sig/Init _____ Sig/Init _____

Sig/Init _____ Sig/Init _____

Sig/Init _____ Sig/Init _____

FIGURE D.2 Temporary Prescription Log

Workflows

Instructions

The worksheets in this appendix are designed to aid in the transition from a paper-based process to an electronic process.

Figure E.1—E-Rx Implementation Checklist: Users can adapt this tool to fit their needs, according to the vendor with whom they are working. Having a checklist ensures critical steps are completed before using the application in a live environment.

Figure E.2—Preimplementation and Postimplementation Workflows: These tools address nonprescribing workflow needs. E-prescribing may shift work within an office. This tool helps to identify where that shifting will occur and what resources will be needed.

Figures E.3 through E.8—Prescribing Workflows: The way new prescriptions and renewal requests are handled may be very different in a paper environment as opposed to an electronic environment. These worksheets depict common workflows for these processes. The office managers or prescribers can use the blank template in Figure E.3 to diagram their own processes, both before and after implementation. This helps to focus on barriers to the implementation process, if any. In addition, it is a useful tool for communication with others as to what the new workflows will be.

Figures E.9 through E.12—Sample Renewal Workflows: These sample workflows represent the process one office used to determine the roles played by the staff according to the various ways renewal requests could enter the medical office.

E-Rx Implementation Checklist

☐ **Hardware present**
- ◦ For prescribers
- ◦ For nurses
- ◦ For support staff

☐ **Internet access**
- ◦ For prescribers
- ◦ For nurses
- ◦ For support staff

☐ **Printer available for prescriptions**

☐ **Ordered prescription paper for printer**

☐ **Workflows completed**
- ◦ For new prescriptions
- ◦ For renewal requests
- ◦ For disaster plan
- ◦ For reports
- ◦ For data entry
- ◦ For patient education (optional)

☐ Demographics loaded

☐ Training completed
- ◦ For prescribers
- ◦ For nurses
- ◦ For support staff

☐ Critical medication histories loaded

☐ Go live!

Notes:

FIGURE E.1 E-Rx Implementation Checklist

Supporting Workflow Questions—**Before Implementation**

Data Entry (patient demographics and medication histories)

Where are patient problems/ diagnoses updated? What percent of the time?

☐ Exam room ____%
☐ Front office ____%
☐ Central station ____%
☐ Other: _____ ____%

Who records the patient's OTC meds in the chart? What percent of the time?

☐ Prescriber ____%
☐ Nurse ____%
☐ Assistant ____%
☐ Other: _____ ____%

Who updates patient demographics in the chart? What percent of the time?

☐ Prescriber ____%
☐ Nurse ____%
☐ Assistant ____%
☐ Other: _____ ____%

Who records the patient's pharmacy insurance coverage (if done)?

☐ Prescriber
☐ Nurse
☐ Assistant
☐ Other: _____

Who records the patient's active medication history in the chart? What percent of the time?

☐ Prescriber ____%
☐ Nurse ____%
☐ Assistant ____%
☐ Other: _____ ____%

Who records the patient's pharmacy preference (if done)?

☐ Prescriber
☐ Nurse
☐ Assistant
☐ Other: _____

Patient Education/Tools

Who readies prescriptions for authorizing? What percent of the time?

☐ Prescriber ____%
☐ Nurse ____%
☐ Assistant ____%
☐ Other: _____ ____%

Who provides the patient with a current list of his or her medications (if done)?

☐ Prescriber
☐ Nurse
☐ Assistant
☐ Other: _____

FIGURE E.2 Supporting Workflow Questions—Before and After Implementation

Supporting Workflow Questions—**After Implementation**

Data Entry (patient demographics and medication histories)

Where do you expect the eRx application to be used? What percent of the time?

☐ Exam room _____%
☐ Front office _____%
☐ Central station _____%
☐ Other: _____ _____%

Who will enter the patient's OTC meds? What percent of the time?

☐ Prescriber _____%
☐ Nurse _____%
☐ Assistant _____%
☐ Other: _____ _____%

Who will enter demographics? What percent of the time?

☐ Prescriber _____%
☐ Nurse _____%
☐ Assistant _____%
☐ Other: _____ _____%

Who updates the patient's pharmacy information?

☐ Prescriber
☐ Nurse
☐ Assistant
☐ Other: _____

Who will enter the patient's active medication history? What percent of the time?

☐ Prescriber _____%
☐ Nurse _____%
☐ Assistant _____%
☐ Other: _____ _____%

Who records the pharmacy insurance information?

☐ Prescriber
☐ Nurse
☐ Assistant
☐ Other: _____

Patient Education/Tools

Who will retrieve prescriptions from the printer for authorizing? What percent of the time?

☐ Prescriber _____%
☐ Nurse _____%
☐ Assistant _____%
☐ Other: _____ _____%

Who will provide the patient with a current list of his or her medications (if done)?

☐ Prescriber
☐ Nurse
☐ Assistant
☐ Other: _____

FIGURE E.2 (continued)

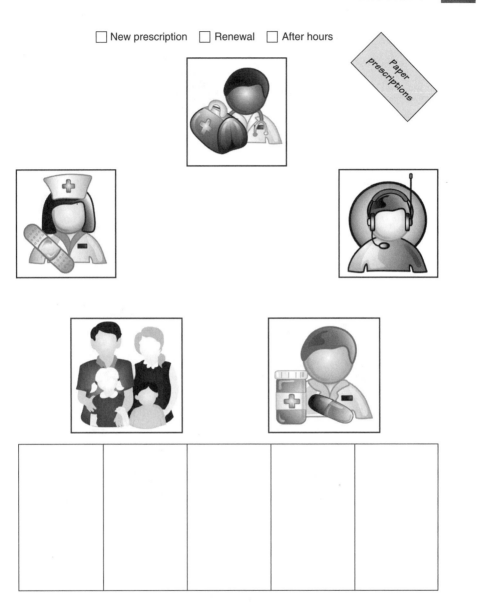

FIGURE E.3 Blank eRx Workflow Template

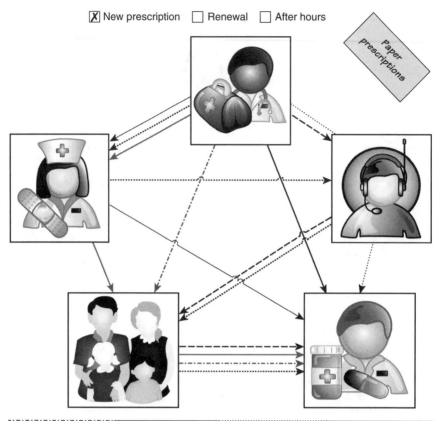

FIGURE E.4 New Paper Prescription Workflow

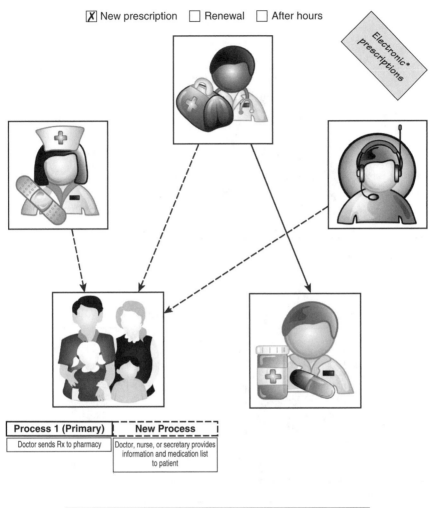

FIGURE E.5 New e-Prescription Workflow

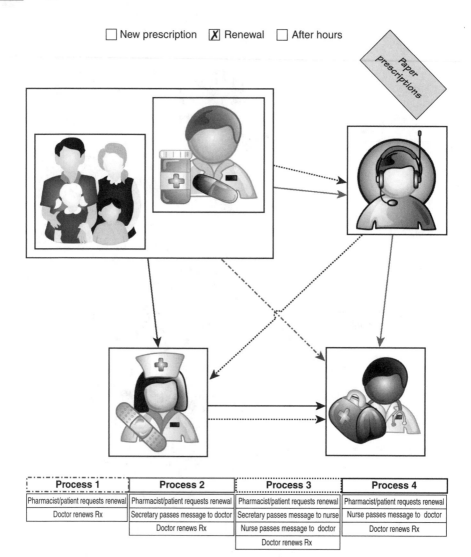

☐ New prescription   ☒ Renewal   ☐ After hours

Process 1	Process 2	Process 3	Process 4
Pharmacist/patient requests renewal	Pharmacist/patient requests renewal	Pharmacist/patient requests renewal	Pharmacist/patient requests renewal
Doctor renews Rx	Secretary passes message to doctor	Secretary passes message to nurse	Nurse passes message to doctor
	Doctor renews Rx	Nurse passes message to doctor	Doctor renews Rx
		Doctor renews Rx	

FIGURE E.6 Renewal Request for Paper Prescription

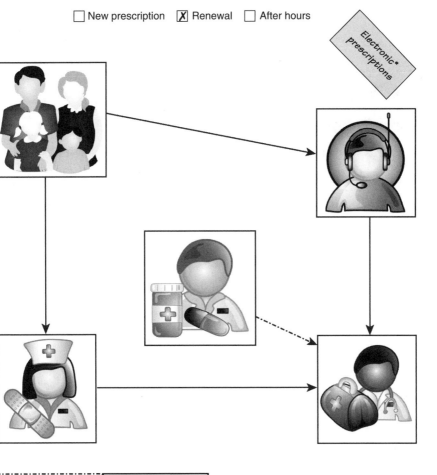

☐ New prescription   ☒ Renewal   ☐ After hours

Electronic * Prescriptions

Process 1	Process 2
Pharmacist requests e-renewal	Patient requests renewal
Doctor renews Rx	Nurse/secretary renews Rx
	Doctor authorizes Rx

*When prescriptions must be printed, they follow the same flows as paper prescriptions.

FIGURE E.7 Renewal Request for e-Prescription

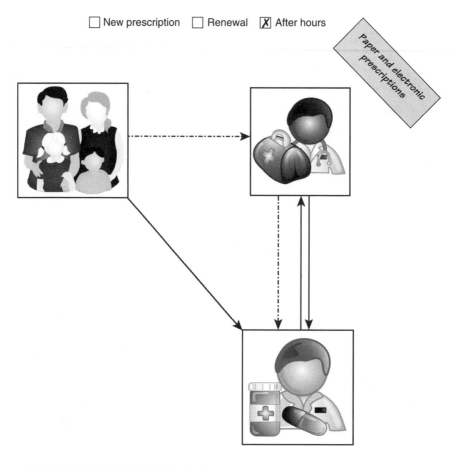

☐ New prescription ☐ Renewal ☒ After hours

Paper and electronic prescriptions

Process 1	Process 2
Patient reaches on call doctor	Patient goes to pharmacy
Doctor phones/sends Rx to pharmacy	Pharmacist reaches on call doctor
	Doctor phones/sends Rx to pharmacy

FIGURE E.8 After-Hours Workflow

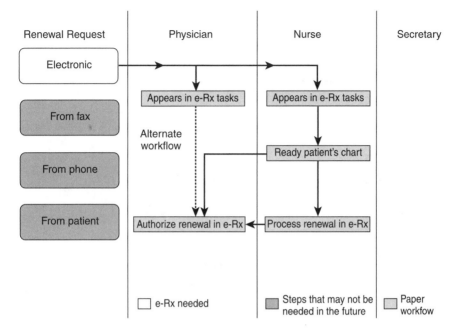

FIGURE E.9 Renewal Workflow from Pharmacy

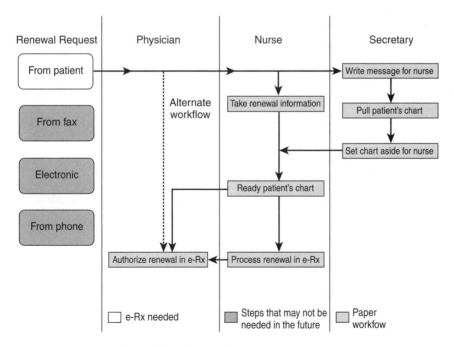

FIGURE E.10 Renewal Workflow from Patient

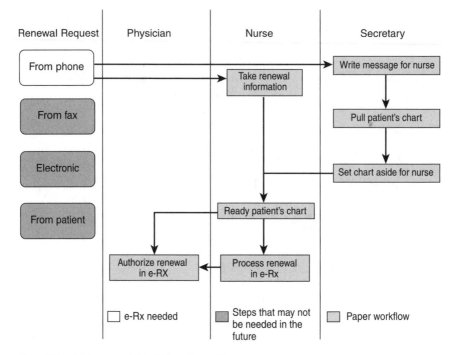

FIGURE E.11 Renewal Workflow from Phone

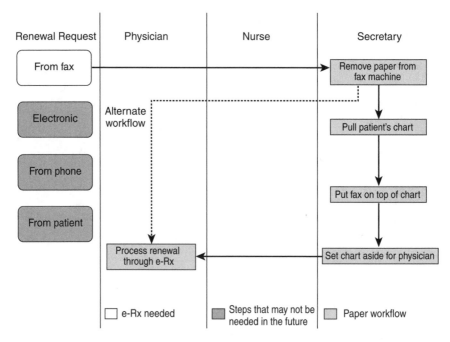

FIGURE E.12 Renewal Workflow from Fax

Training

Figure F.1 depicts a training sheet that can be adapted for use when training basic features of an e-prescribing application. The instructor can use the checkboxes to ensure the material is covered, while the exercises below can be checked by the student as they are completed. This provides a balance between didactic teaching and supervised practice during the training session. **Figure F.2** covers the learning areas pertinent to prescribing, and **Figure F.3** covers the learning areas pertinent to administrators.

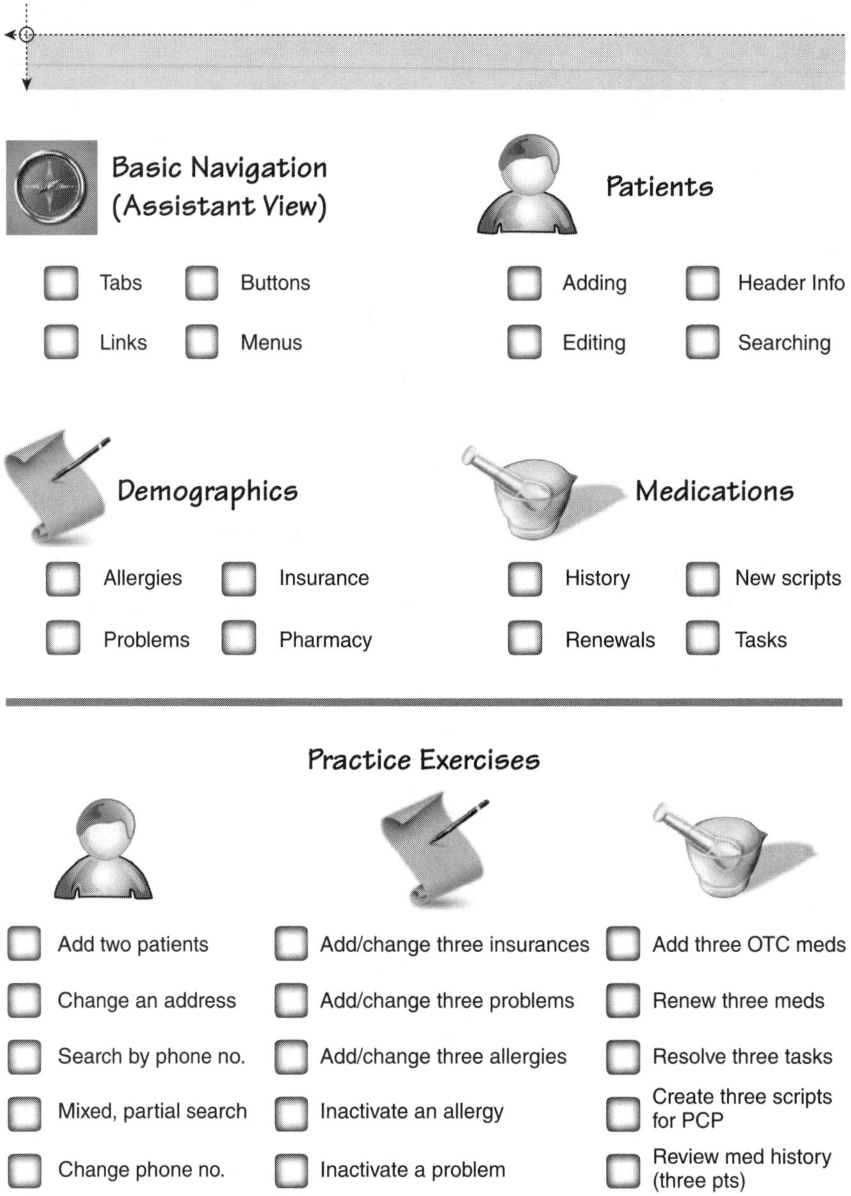

Basic Navigation (Assistant View)

☐ Tabs ☐ Buttons
☐ Links ☐ Menus

Patients

☐ Adding ☐ Header Info
☐ Editing ☐ Searching

Demographics

☐ Allergies ☐ Insurance
☐ Problems ☐ Pharmacy

Medications

☐ History ☐ New scripts
☐ Renewals ☐ Tasks

Practice Exercises

☐ Add two patients
☐ Change an address
☐ Search by phone no.
☐ Mixed, partial search
☐ Change phone no.

☐ Add/change three insurances
☐ Add/change three problems
☐ Add/change three allergies
☐ Inactivate an allergy
☐ Inactivate a problem

☐ Add three OTC meds
☐ Renew three meds
☐ Resolve three tasks
☐ Create three scripts for PCP
☐ Review med history (three pts)

FIGURE F.1 E-Rx Training Checklist—Core Session

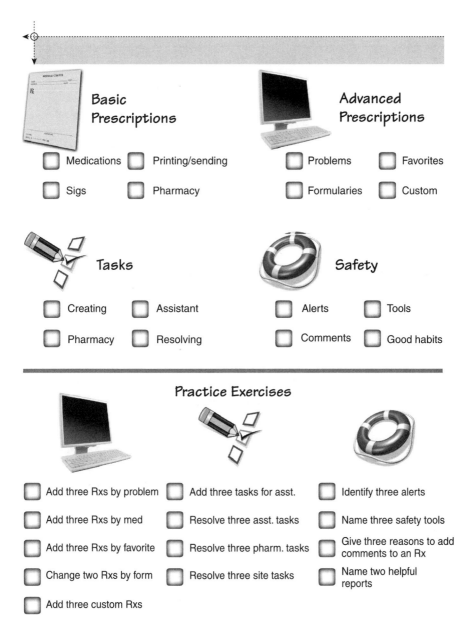

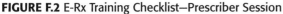

FIGURE F.2 E-Rx Training Checklist—Prescriber Session

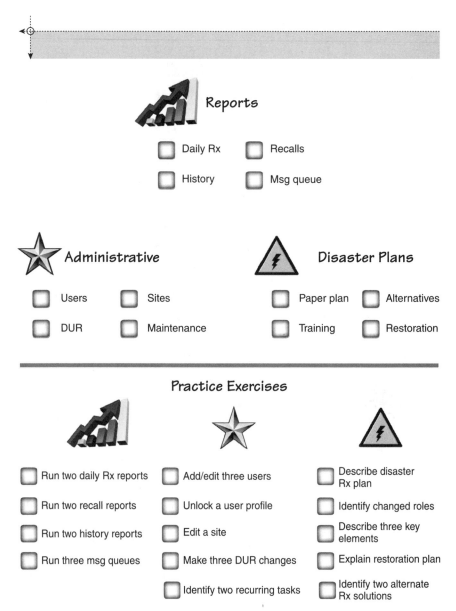

FIGURE F.3 E-Rx Training Checklist—Advanced Session

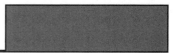

Glossary

Allscripts The vendor for the e-prescribing program, eRx NOW. See also www.allscripts.com.

Application elements The various components and discrete functions of an application such as the user interface, drug selection screens, and clinical alert settings.

Clinical decision support (CDS) Computer tools or applications to assist physicians in clinical decisions by providing evidence-based knowledge in the context of patient-specific data. Examples include drug interaction alerts at the time medication is prescribed and reminders for specific guideline-based interventions during the care of patients with chronic disease. Information should be presented in a patient-centric view of individual care and also in a population or aggregate view to support population management and quality improvement.[22]

CMS An abbreviation for Centers for Medicaid and Medicare Services.

Dispenser A person or other legal entity, licensed, registered, or otherwise permitted by the jurisdiction in which the person practices or the entity is located, to provide drug products for human use by prescription in the course of professional practice.[50]

Drug utilization review (DUR) A system of drug use review that can identify potential adverse drug interactions, drug-condition conflicts, therapeutic duplication, drug–age conflicts, etc. There are three forms of drug utilization checks: prospective (which takes place before prescription dispensing), concurrent (which takes place at the time of dispensing), and retrospective (which takes place after the therapy has been completed). Appropriate use of an integrated drug-utilization check program can curb drug misuse and abuse and monitor quality of care. This safety measure can reduce hospitalization and other costs related to inappropriate drug use.[23]

Electronic data interchange (EDI) A set of standards for structuring information that is to be electronically exchanged between and within businesses, organizations, government entities, and other groups.[131]

Electronic health record (EHR) A real-time patient health record with access to evidence-based decision support tools that can be used to aid clinicians in decision making. The EHR can automate and streamline a clinician's workflow, ensuring that all clinical information is communicated. It can also prevent delays in response that result in gaps in care. The EHR can also support the collection of data for uses other than clinical care, such as billing, quality management, outcome reporting, and public health disease surveillance and reporting.[22]

Electronic media Electronic storage media including memory devices in computers (hard drives), and any removable/transportable digital memory medium, such as magnetic tape or disk, optical disk, or digital memory card; or transmission media used to exchange information already in electronic storage media. Transmission media include, for example, the internet (wide open), extranet (using internet technology to link a business with information only accessible to collaborating parties), leased lines, dial-up lines, private networks, and the physical movement of removable/transportable electronic storage media. Certain transmissions, including of paper, via facsimile, and of voice, via telephone, are not considered to be transmissions via electronic media, because the information being exchanged did not exist in electronic form before the transmission.[50]

Electronic medical record (EMR) This technology, when fully developed, meets provider needs for real-time data access and evaluation in medical care. In concert with clinical workstations, point-of-care devices, and clinical data repository technologies, the EMR provides the means for longitudinal data storage and access.[23]

Electronic prescribing (e-prescribing, e-Rx) The transmission, using electronic media, of prescription or prescription-related information, between a prescriber, dispenser, PBM, or health plan, either directly or through an intermediary, including an e-prescribing network.[50]

Electronic prescription (e-prescription) Refers to prescription information that is created, stored, and transmitted via electronic means by computer or handheld device. The term *electronic prescriptions* does not apply to prescriptions communicated either by facsimile (fax) or over the phone.[23]

eRx NOW The e-prescribing application created by Allscripts and made freely available through NEPSI in February of 2007.

Final standards Uniform standards that are adopted through notice and comment rule making for use in the e-prescribing program under Title I of the MMA. Medicare prescription drug program sponsors, Medicare Advantage (MA) organizations offering Medicare Advantage prescription drug (MA-PD) plans, and other Part D sponsors will be required to support and comply with these standards when electronically transmitting prescriptions and prescription-related information between dispensing pharmacies and pharmacists.[24]

Formulary A list of preferred medications. It is used as a mechanism to encourage the use of less-costly drugs. Formularies should be updated frequently to reflect new drugs being introduced into the market, current clinical information, and information on drug interactions.[23]

Foundation standards Standards for which there is adequate industry experience that have been adopted by the DHHS secretary through notice and comment rule making without pilot testing.[24]

Healthcare information exchange (HIE) A multi-stakeholder entity that enables the movement of health-related data within state, regional, or non-jurisdictional participant groups.[97]

HL-7 (Health Level 7) One of several American National Standards Institute-accredited standards developing organizations operating in the healthcare arena. Most standards-developing organizations produce standards (sometimes called specifications or protocols) for a particular healthcare domain such as pharmacy, medical devices, imaging, or insurance (claims processing) transactions. Health Level 7's domain is clinical and administrative data.[69]

ICD-9 The *International Classification of Diseases* (ICD), ninth revision, is designed to promote international comparability in the collection, processing, classification, and presentation of mortality statistics. See also www.cdc.gov/nchs/about/major/dvs/icd9des.htm.

Initial standards NCVHS reviewed and commented on standards that were ultimately recognized by the secretary as initial uniform standards relating to the requirements for e-prescribing. These standards lacked adequate industry experience and thus were subject to pilot testing via the AHRQ interagency agreement with CMS.[24]

Integrated application A healthcare application that communicates with data sources to provide enhanced functionality. For example, an EMR receives laboratory data from the local health system, or an e-prescribing application receives patient demographic updates and medication history from an HIE.

Interface The code written and the specifications and protocols used for the electronic data exchange between the participants' and/or vendors' computing environments.[23]

JITI An acronym for just-in-time information. In this book, JITI includes clinical information (e.g., interaction alerts, drug information), economic information (e.g., formulary alerts, patient co-pays), and workflow information (e.g., role support, context-sensitive application elements).

Master patient or **member index (MPI** or **MMI)** An index or file with a unique identifier for each patient or member that serves as a key to a patient's or member's health record.[23]

Medication error Any error occurring in the medication use process. Includes preventable, inappropriate use of medication including prescribing, dispensing, and administering.[24]

Medication history (Hx) An electronic standard that includes the status, provider, patient, coordination of benefit, repeatable drug, request, and response segments of SCRIPT.[24]

National Council for Prescription Drug Programs (NCPDP) A not-for-profit American National Standards Institute–accredited standards development organization that develops and maintains standards through a consensus-building process among more than 1,450 members representing all pharmacy sectors.[24] See also www.ncpdp.org.

National provider identifier (NPI) Widely accepted as the dispenser (pharmacy) identifier (there is currently no single identifier required for prescribers). Its database contains information to support various claims-processing functions.[24]

NCPDP SCRIPT cancellation (CANRX) Cancels a prescription previously sent to a pharmacy.[24]

NCPDP SCRIPT change request and response (RXCHG) The primary means by which a pharmacy may request of a provider a clarification, correction, or change in drug as a result of therapeutic substitution or other rationale.[24]

NCPDP SCRIPT standard (SCRIPT) Provides for the exchange of new prescriptions, changes, renewals, cancellations, change responses, and fill status notifications.[24]

NEPSI An acronym for the National e-Prescribing Patient Safety Initiative.[3]

NSAIDs An acronym for nonsteroidal anti-inflammatory drugs such as naproxen and ibuprofen.

Patient's profile A collection of patient-specific information including demographics, allergies, problems, and medications in the context of e-prescribing or pharmacy dispensing applications.

Pharmacy benefits managers (PBMs) Private companies that administer pharmacy benefits and manage the purchasing, dispensing, and reimbursing of prescription drugs. PBMs provide a wide array of services to health insurers or to large healthcare purchasers and may negotiate rebates or discounts from pharmaceutical manufacturers and retail pharmacies and process claims for prescription drugs. PBMs play a key role in managing pharmacy benefit plans in the Medicare drug program.[24]

Practice management system (PMS) Tools (usually computer software) that organize routine medical and business tasks.[24]

Prescriber A physician, dentist, or other person licensed, registered, or otherwise permitted by the United States or the jurisdiction in which he or she practices to issue prescriptions for drugs for human use.[24]

Prescription-related information Information regarding eligibility for drug benefits, medication history, or related health or drug information for a Part D–eligible individual enrolled in a Part D plan.[50]

Prior authorization The portion of X12N 278 standard that supports prior authorization. It requires header information, requester, subscriber, utilization management, and other relevant information.[24]

Regional health information organization (RHIO) A group of organizations with a business stake in improving the quality, safety, and efficiency of healthcare delivery.[132]

RxHub An organization founded in 2001 by the three leading pharmacy benefit managers (PBMs): AdvancePCS, Express Scripts, and Medco Health Solutions. RxHub is connecting the industry to electronically route up-to-date patient medication history and pharmacy benefit information to physicians in their offices and at hospitals. See also www.rxhub.net.

RxNorm A clinical drug nomenclature produced by the National Library of Medicine that provides standard names for clinical drugs and for dose forms, and links from clinical drugs to their active ingredients, drug components, and most related brand names. It includes the semantic clinical drug (ingredient plus strength and dose form) and the semantic branded drug representation (proprietary, branded ingredient plus strength).[24]

Schedule II drugs A drug or chemical substance whose possession and use are regulated under the Controlled Substances Act, including, among others, narcotics and hallucinogens.[24]

Sig Latin abbreviation for *signa,* which means write or label. In the context of prescriptions, it denotes the content of patient instructions to be printed on the container of the dispensed medication.

SureScripts An organization founded in 2001 by the National Association of Chain Drug Stores (NACDS) and the National Community Pharmacists Association (NCPA). The Pharmacy Health Information Exchange, operated by SureScripts, is the largest network to link electronic communications between pharmacies and physicians, allowing the electronic exchange of prescription information.[133]

Vendor A company that sells a product. In this book, the product is most frequently an electronic prescribing program or pharmacy dispensing program.

X12N 270/271 The HIPAA standard for eligibility and benefits communications between dentists, professionals, institutions, and health plans.[24]

References

1. Ash JS, Sittig DF, Poon EG. The extent and importance of unintended consequences related to computerized provider order entry. J Am Med Inform Assoc 2007 July/Aug; 14 (4): 415–23

2. IOM. To err is human: building a safer health system. Washington (DC): National Academies Press, 1999

3. NEPSI. National eprescribing patient safety initiative. Available from URL: http://www.nationalerx.com/ [Accessed 2007 May 20]

4. Ferner RE. Commentary: computer aided prescribing leaves holes in the safety net. Br Med J 2004, May 15; 328: 1172–3

5. Shamliyan TA, Duval S, Du J, et al. Just what the doctor ordered. Review of the evidence of the impact of computerized physician order entry system on medication errors. Health Serv Res 2007, June 26: 1–22

6. Tom WC. New developments for electronic prescribing. Pharmacist's Letter/Prescriber's Letter 2007 March; 23 (230301): 1–5

7. Rupp M. E-prescribing: the value proposition. America's Pharmacist 2005, Apr: 23–6

8. Rupp M. The impact of e-prescribing on staff productivity in community pharmacy—Part 2. Comput Talk 2005; 25 (4): 14–7

9. Rupp M. The impact of e-prescribing on staff productivity in community pharmacy—Part 1. Comput Talk 2005; 25 (3): 15–22

10. ISMP. A call to action: eliminate handwritten prescriptions within 3 years! [white paper] 2000; 1–13. Available from URL: http://www.ismp.org/Newsletters/acutecare/articles/Whitepaper.asp [Accessed 2007 May 19]

11. Aspden P, Wolcott JA, Bootman L, et al. for the Institute of Medicine. Preventing medication errors. Washington (DC): National Academies Press, 2007

12. Fortescue EB, Kaushal R, McKenna K. Prioritizing strategies for preventing medication errors and adverse drug events in pediatric inpatients. Pediatrics 2003 Apr; 111, (4): 722–30

13. Tamblyn R, Huang A, Kawasumi Y. The development and evaluation of an integrated electronic prescribing and drug management system for primary care. J Am Med Inform Assoc 2006 March/Apr; 13 (2): 48–59

14. Buckley M. Improving drug prescribing practices in the outpatient setting: a market analysis. California HealthCare Foundation 2002 Oct: 1–37

15. Lehmann CU, Kim GR. Prevention of medication errors. Clin Perinatol 2005; 32: 107–23

16. Weant KA, Cook AM, Armistead JA. Medication-error reporting and pharmacy resident experience during implementation of computerized prescriber order entry. Am J Health Syst Pharm 2007 Mar 1; 64: 526–30

17. Bobb A, Gleason K, Husch M, et al. The epidemiology of prescribing errors. Arch Intern Med 2004 Apr 12; 164: 785–92

18. Grossman JM, Gerland A, Reed MC, et al. Physician's experiences using commercial e-prescribing systems. Health Affairs—web exclusive 2007 Apr 3; 26 (3): w393–w404

19. Grout J. Mistake-proofing the design of health care processes. Rockville (MD): Agency for Healthcare Research and Quality, 2007

20. Dykes PC, Hurley A, Cashen M. Development and psychometric evaluation of the impact of health information technology (I-HIT) scale. J Am Med Inform Assoc 2007 July/Aug;14 (4): 507–14

21. Eslami S, Abu-Hanna A, DeKeizer NF. Evaluation of outpatient computerized physician medication order entry systems: a systematic review. J Am Med Inform Assoc 2007 July/Aug; 14 (4): 400–6

22. DHHS. Glossary of selected [health information] terms, 2004 Nov. Available from URL: http://www.hhs.gov/healthit/glossary.html [Accessed 2007 Oct 11]

23. RxHub. Resource center—glossary, 2007. Available from URL: http://www.rxhub.net/index.php?option=com_content&task=view&id=3 6&Itemid=47 [Accessed 2008 Jan 23]

24. Leavitt MO. Pilot testing of initial electronic prescribing standards—cooperative agreements required under section 1860D-(4)(e) of the Social Security Act as amended by the Medicare Prescription Drug, Improvement, and Modernization Action (MMA) of 2003. Washington (DC): Centers for Medicare and Medicaid Services, 2007

25. Health Insurance Portability and Accountability Act (HIPAA) of 1996. Public Law No 104–191, 110 Stat 1936; 1996

26. Greenberg MD, Ridgely MS, Bell DS. Electronic prescribing and HIPAA privacy regulation. Inquiry 2004/2005 Winter; 41: 461–8

27. SureScripts. Get your practice connected, 2007. Available from URL: http://www.surescripts.com/get-connected.aspx?ptype=physician [Accessed 2007 May 19]

28. CMS. Medicare program; [...] the amendment of the e-prescribing exemption for computer-generated facsimile transmissions. Federal Register Nov 27 2007: 66334–66339

29. Classen D, Pestotnik SL, Evans S, et al. Adverse drug events in hospitalized patients. JAMA 1997; 227: 301–6

30. Bates DW, Spell N, Cullen DJ, et al. The costs of adverse drug events in hospitalized patients. JAMA 1997; 277: 307–11

31. Birkmeyer CM, Lee J, Bates DW, et al. Will electronic order entry reduce health care costs? Eff Clin Pract 2002 Mar/Apr; 5: 67–74

32. IOM. Preventing medication errors [report brief], 2006 July. Available from URL: http://www.iom.edu/CMS/3809/22526/35939/35943.aspx [Accessed 2007 May 19]

33. JCAHO. FAQs for the Joint Commission's 2007 national patient safety goals, 2007 Jan. Available from URL: http://www.jointcommission.org/ NR/rdonlyres/9ECF1ED6-E04E-41DE-B7BC-174590CEDF33/0/07_ NPSG_FAQs_8.pdf [Accessed 2007 May 19]

34. FY 2008 performance budget, Drug Enforcement Administration, congressional budget submission. Alexandria (VA): Drug Enforcement Administration; 2007: DEA-107

35. Electronic prescriptions for controlled substances (EPCS). Alexandria (VA): Drug Enforcement Administration; 2006

36. New York State Education Department, Office of the Professions. Current issues in pharmacy, 2006 Nov 7. Available from URL: http://www.op. nysed.gov/pharmelectrans.htm [Accessed 2008 Feb 6]

37. Whitehouse S. Whitehouse chairs hearing to investigate barrier to e-prescribing, 2007 Dec 4. Available from URL: http://www.whitehouse. senate.gov/record.cfm?id=288248& [Accessed 2007 Dec 4]

38. Hale PL, editor. Electronic prescribing for the medical practice: everything you wanted to know but were afraid to ask. Chicago (IL): HIMSS, 2007

39. Shah SNH, Aslam M, Avery AJ. A survey of prescription errors in general practice. Pharm J 2001 Dec 15; 267: 860-2

40. Kilbridge PM, Classen D, Bates DW, et al. The national quality form safe practice standard for computerized physician order entry: updating a critical patient safety practice. J Patient Safety 2006 Dec; 2 (4): 183–90

41. Cohen M, editor. Medication errors. Washington (DC): American Pharmaceutical Association, 1999

42. Horsky J, Kuperman GJ, Patel VL. Comprehensive analysis of a medication dosing error related to CPOE. J Am Med Inform Assoc 2005 Jul–Aug; 12 (4): 377–82

43. Gandhi TK, Weingart SN, Seger AC, et al. Outpatient prescribing errors and the impact of computerized prescribing. J Gen Intern Med 2005; 20: 837–41

44. Welch WP, Bazarko D, Ritten K. Electronic health records in four community physician practices: impact on quality and cost of care. J Am Med Inform Assoc 2007 June, 14 (3): 320–8

45. Walsh KE, Kaushal R, Chessare JB. How to avoid paediatric medication errors: a user's guide to the literature. Br Med J 2005 Nov 7: 698–702

46. Blum KV, Urbanski CJ, Pierce JM. Medication error prevention by pharmacists. Am J Hosp Pharm 1988 Sept; 45:1902–3

47. Raebel MA, Charles J, Dugan J, et al. Randomized trial to improve prescribing safety in ambulatory elderly patients. J Am Geriatr Soc 2007; 55: 977–85

48. SureScripts. SureScripts home page, 2007. Available from URL: http://www.surescripts.com/Default.aspx [Accessed 2007 May 19]

49. Hollingworth W, Devine EB, Hansen RN, et al. The impact of e-prescribing on prescriber and staff time in ambulatory care clinics: a time motion study. J Am Med Inform Assoc 2007 Nov–Dec; 14(6): 722–30

50. CMS. Medicare program; e-prescribing and the prescription drug program; final rule. Federal Register 2005: 67568-95

51. Perlin JB, Gelinas LS. Draft letter Electronic Health Records Work Group to Michael Leavitt, American Health Information Community Chairman, 2007 Nov 26. Available from URL: http://www.hhs.gov/healthit/documents/m20071128/letter.html [Accessed 2007 December 4th]

52. Bell DS. Pilot testing of electronic prescribing standards. Rockville (MD): Agency for Healthcare Research and Quality, 2007 Jan 31; Grant No.: 1U18HS016391-01

53. CMS. Medicare program; proposed standards for e-prescribing under Medicare Part D. Federal Register 2007 Nov 16: 64900-18

54. APHA. Statement of the American Pharmacists Association on electronic prescribing of controlled substances: addressing health care and law enforcement priorities. Washington (DC): American Pharmacists Association, 2007 Dec 4.

55. RxHub. About RxHub, 2007. Available from URL: http://www.rxhub.net/index.php?option=com_content&task=view&id=28&Itemid=39 [Accessed 2008 Jan 23]

56. AHIP. Innovations in health information technology, 2005; Chapter 2. Available from URL: http://www.ahipresearch.org/pdfs/AHIP_InvHealthIT_05.pdf [Accessed 2007 May 20]

57. Teich J, Osheroff J, Pifer E, et al. Clinical decision support in electronic prescribing: recommendations and an action plan. J Am Med Inform Assoc 2005; 12: 365–76

58. Warholak-Juarez T, Rupp M. The effect of patient information on the quality of pharmacists' drug use review decisions. J Am Pharm Assoc 2000; 40: 500–8

59. NCPDP. NCPDP home page, 2007. [Home page for the e-prescribing standards-setting organization]. Available from URL: http://www.ncpdp. org/ [Accessed 2007 Aug 4]

60. eRx Network: company overview, 2007. Available from URL: http://www. erxnetwork.com/CompanyOverview.aspx [Accessed 2007 Nov 23]

61. RelayHealth. About RelayHealth, 2007. Available from URL: https:// www.relayhealth.com/rh/general/aboutUs/default.aspx [Accessed 2007 Nov 23]

62. RelayHealth. McKesson welcomes Per-Se, announces new connectivity business, 2007. Available from URL: https://www.relayhealth.com/rh/ general/news/newsRecent/news105.aspx [Accessed 2007 Nov 23]

63. Miller RA, Gardner RM, Johnson K, et al. Clinical decision support and electronic prescribing systems: a time for responsible thought and action. J Am Med Inform Assoc 2005 July/Aug; 12 (4): 403–9

64. Van der Sijs H, Aarts J, Vulto A, et al. Overriding of drug safety alerts in computerized physician order entry. J Am Med Inform Assoc 2006; 13: 138–47

65. Steele AW, Eisert S, Witter J. The effect of automated alerts on provider ordering behavior in an outpatient setting. PLoS Med 2005 Sept; 2 (9): 864–70

66. Judge J, Field TS, DeFlorio M. Prescribers' responses to alerts during medication ordering in the long term care setting. J Am Med Inform Assoc 2006 July/Aug; 13 (4): 385–90

67. Weingart SN, Toth M, Sands DZ. Physicians' decisions to override computerized drug alerts in primary care. Arch Intern Med 2003 Nov 24; 163: 2625–31

68. National Library of Medicine. Unified medical language system: RxNorm, 2004 [resource for RxNorm information]. Available from URL: http://www.nlm.nih.gov/research/umls/rxnorm/index.html [Accessed 2007 Aug 4th]

69. HL-7. HL-7 home page, 2007 Aug 2. Available from URL: http://www. hl7.org/ [Accessed 2007 Aug 4]

70. HL-7, NCPDP. NCPDP-HL7 electronic prescribing coordination mapping document [draft release]; 2005. Report No. 1.0

71. Wang CJ, Marken RS, Meili RC, et al. Functional characteristics of commercial ambulatory electronic prescribing systems: a field study. J Am Med Inform Assoc 2005; 12: 346–56

72. Pifer E. CPOE-related errors: what can the literature teach us about designing and using these systems? Healthc Inform 2005 Aug: 1197–203

73. Miller AS. Pharmacy issues: clinical screenings and discharge prescriptions. Hosp Pharm 2001; 36 (12): 1290–5

74. Weingart SN, Hamrick HE, Tutkus S. Medication safety messages for patients via the web portal: the MedCheck intervention. Int J Med Inform 2007 Jun 18; 77 (3): 161-8. Epub 2007 Jun 19

75. Kuperman GJ, Bobb A, Payne T, et al. Medication-related clinical decision support in computerized provider order entry systems: a review. J Am Med Inform Assoc 2007; 14 (1): 29–49

76. Kuperman GJ, Gandhi TK, Bates DW. Effective drug-allergy checking: methodological and operational issues. J Biomed Inform 2003; 36: 70–9

77. Abookire SA, Teich J, Sandige H, et al. Improving allergy alerting in a computerized physician order entry system. AMIA; 2000: 2–6

78. Hsieh TC, Kuperman GJ, Jaggi T, et al. Characteristics and consequences of drug allergy alert overrides in a computerized physician order entry system. J Am Med Inform Assoc 2004; 11: 482–91

79. NHLBI. Guidelines for the diagnosis and management of asthma. Department of Health and Human Services 1997: 123

80. JCAHO. Implementation tips for eliminating dangerous abbreviations; 2007 Jan. Available from URL: http://www.jointcommission.org/PatientSafety/NationalPatientSafetyGoals/abbr_tips.htm [Accessed 2007 May 19]

81. Demiris G, Afrin LB, Speedie S, et al. Patient-centered applications: use of information technology to promote disease management and wellness. J Am Med Inform Assoc 2007 Oct 18 [Preprint doi:10.1197/jamia. M2492]

82. Nissen SE, Wolski K. Effect of rosiglitazone on the risk of myocardial infarction and death from cardiovascular causes. N Engl J Med 2007 June 14; 356 (24): 2457–71

83. Orlowski JP, Wateska L. The effects of pharmaceutical firm enticements on physician prescribing patterns. Chest 1992; 102: 270–73

84. Caudill TS, Johnson MS, Rich EC, et al. Physicians, pharmaceutical sales representatives and the cost of prescribing. Arch Fam Med 1996; 5: 201–6

85. Symm B, Averitt M, Forjuoh SN, et al. Effects of using free sample medications on prescribing practices of family physicians. J Am Board Fam Med 2006; 19 (5): 443–9

86. Chew LD, O'Young TS, Hazlet TK, et al. A physician survey of the effect of drug sample availability on physicians' behavior. J Gen Intern Med 2000; 15: 478–83

87. Adair RF, Holmgren LR. Do drug samples influence resident prescribing behavior? A randomized trial. Am J Med 2005; 118: 881–4

88. Haller G, Myles PS, Stoelwinder J. Integrating incident reporting into an electronic patient record system. J Am Med Inform Assoc 2007; March/Apr; 14 (2): 175–81

89. HIMSS. Identifying stakeholders and goals; improving outcomes with clinical decision support: an implementer's guide. Chicago (IL): HIMSS, 2004: 1–23

90. Javitt JC, Steinberg G, Locke T. Using a claims data-based sentinel system to improve compliance with clinical guidelines: results of a randomized prospective study. Am J Manag Care 2005 Feb; 11 (2): 93–102

91. Kaelber DC, Bates DW. Health information exchange and patient safety. J Biomed Inform 2007; doi:10.1016/j.jbi.2007.08.011

92. Wright A, Goldberg H, Hongsermeier T. A description and functional taxonomy of rule-based decision support content at a large integrated delivery network. J Am Med Inform Assoc 2007 July/Aug; 14 (4): 489–96

93. Juster IA. Technology-driven interactive care management identifies and resolves more clinical issues than a claims-based alerting system. Technology-Driven Interactive Care Management 2005; 8 (3): 188–97

94. Glassman PA, Belperio P, Lanto A. The utility of adding retrospective medication profiling to computerized provider order entry in an ambulatory care population. J Am Med Inform Assoc 2007 Aug; 14 (4): 424–31

95. Baron RJ. Quality improvement with an electronic health record: achievable, but not automatic. Ann Intern Med 2007; 147: 549–52

96. Jaski ME, Schwartzberg J, Guttman RA. Medication review and documentation in physician office practice. Eff Clin Pract 2000 Jan/Feb; 3 (1): 30–4

97. DHHS. Medication management: detailed use case. Washington (DC): Department of Health and Human Services, 2007: 47

98. Pifer E. The impact of clinical decision support systems: alerts and standardized order sets. Institute for Safe Medication Practices Teleconference; 2006 June 29

99. Shah SNH, Seger AC, Seger DL, et al. Improving acceptance of computerized prescribing alerts in ambulatory care. J Am Med Inform Assoc 2006; 13 (1): 5–11

100. Spina JR, Glassman PA, Belperio P, et al. Clinical relevance of automated drug alerts from the perspective of medical providers. Am J Med Qual 2005 Jan/Feb; 20 (1): 7–14

101. Solberg LI. Measuring patient safety in ambulatory care: potential for identifying medical group drug–drug interaction rates using claims data. Am J Manag Care 2004 Nov; 10 (11): 753–9

102. Feldstein A, Simon SR, Schneider J. How to design computerized alerts to ensure safe prescribing practices. Jt Comm J Qual Saf 2004 Nov; 30 (11): 602–13

103. Payne TH, Nichol WP, Hoey P, et al. Characteristics and override rates of order checks in a practitioner order entry system. Annu Symp Proc. 2002; 602–6

104. Peterson JF, Bates DW. Preventable medication errors: identifying and eliminating serious drug interactions. J Am Pharm Assoc 2001 March/Apr; 41 (2): 159

105. Hickner JM, Fernald D, Harris DM. Issues and initiatives in the testing process in primary care physician offices. Jt Comm J Qual Patient Saf 2005 Feb; 31 (2): 81–9

106. Medication management and polypharmacy: Beer's list, 2002. Available from URL: http://www.tahsa.org/files%2FDDF%2Fmedbeer1.pdf [Accessed 2007 Nov 3]

107. Potentially inappropriate medications for the elderly according to the revised Beers Criteria, 2007. Available from URL: http://www.dcri.duke.edu/ccge/curtis/beers.html [Accessed 2007 Nov 3]

108. Albert KM. Integrating knowledge-based resources into the electronic health record: history, current status, and role of librarians. Med Ref Serv Q 2007; 26 (3): 1–19

109. Schleyer T, Spallek H, Hernandez P. A qualitative investigation of the content of dental paper-based and computer-based patient record formats. J Am Med Inform Assoc 2007 July/Aug;14 (4): 515–26

110. Hoth AB, Carter BL, Ness J. Development and reliability testing of the clinical pharmacist recommendation taxonomy. Pharmacotherapy 2007; 27 (5): 639–46

111. McMurry AJ, Gilbert CA, Reis BY. A self-scaling, distributed information architecture for public health, research, and clinical care. J Am Med Inform Assoc 2007 July/Aug; 14 (4): 527–33

112. Simon JS, Rundall TG, Shortell SM. Adoption of order entry with decision support for chronic care by physician organizations. J Am Med Inform Assoc 2007 July/Aug; 14 (4): 432–9

113. Thomsen LA, Winterstein AG, Sondergaard B, et al. Systematic review of the incidence and characteristics of preventable adverse drug events in ambulatory care. Ann Pharmacother 2007; 41: 1411–26

114. Merck. Merck announces voluntary worldwide withdrawal of Vioxx, 2004. Available from URL: http://www.merck.com/newsroom/vioxx/pdf/vioxx_press_release_final.pdf [Accessed 2007 May 19]

115. JCAHO. Errors associated with new technology. Jt Comm Persp Patient Saf 2007 May; 7 (5): 5–6, 13–4

116. Angell D. HAP, Henry Ford health system e-prescribing technology hits 500,000 'scripts, 2006. Available from URL: http://www.henryfordhealth. org/body.cfm?id=46335&action=detail&ref=560 [Accessed 2007 Nov 7th]

117. ISMP. ISMP's list of confused drug names, 2007. Available from URL: http://www.ismp.org/Tools/confuseddrugnames.pdf [Accessed 2007 Aug 4th]

118. Gurwitz JH, Field TS, Harrold LR, et al. Incidence and preventability of adverse drug events among older persons in the ambulatory setting. JAMA 2003; 289: 1107–16

119. Grizzle AJ, Mahmood MH, Ko Y, et al. Reasons provided by prescribers when overriding drug–drug interaction alerts. Am J Manag Care 2007; 13: 573–80

120. Simon SR, Kaushal R, Cleary PD. Physicians and electronic health records. Arch Intern Med 2007 Mar 12; 167: 507–12

121. Tonkin AL, Taverner D, Latte J. The effect of an interactive tutorial on the prescribing performance of senior medical students. Med Educ Online 2006; 11 (9): 1–6

122. Druskat VU, Wolff SB. Building the emotional intelligence of groups. Har Bus Rev 2001 Mar: 80–90

123. LeTourneau B. Managing physician resistance to change. J Healthc Manag 2004 Sep/Oct; 49 (5): 286–88

124. Gandhi TK, Weingart SN, Borus J, et al. Adverse drug events in ambulatory care. N Engl J Med 2003; 348: 1556–64

125. Woods DD, Cook RI. Mistaking error. In: Youngberg BJ, Hatlie MJ, editors. The patient safety handbook. Sudbury (MA): Jones and Bartlett; 2004

126. Ritzel DO, Saldana MAM, Herrero SG, et al. Assessing definitions and concepts within safety profession. Int Electronic J Health Educ 2003; 6: 1–9

127. Phillips RA, Andrieni JD. Translational patient care: a new model for inpatient care in the 21st century. Arch Intern Med 2007 Oct 22; 167 (19): 2025–6

128. Tam VC, Knowles SR, Cornish PL, et al. Frequency, type and clinical importance of medication history errors at admission to hospital: a systematic review. Can Med Assoc J 2005; 173 (5): 510–5

129. Flabouris A, Runciman WB, Levings B. Incidents during out-of-hospital patient transportation. Anaesth Intensive Care 2006 Apr; 34 (2): 228–36

130. McFadden FR. Six sigma quality programs: an overview of six sigma quality applications for use in the real world. J Qual Prog 1993 Jun; 26 (6): 37–42

131. Wikipedia Contributors. Electronic data interchange, 2007 3 Dec; 23:43 UTC. Available from URL: http://en.wikipedia.org/w/index.php?title= Electronic_Data_Interchange&oldid=175599475 [Accessed 2007 Dec 3]

132. HIMSS. HIMSS RHIO/HIE, 2007. Available from URL: http://www. himss.org/ASP/topics_rhio.asp [Accessed 2008 Feb 12]

133. SureScripts. About SureScripts, 2007. Available from URL: http://www. surescripts.com/SureScripts/about.aspx [Accessed 2008 Feb 12]

Index